Man, Health, and Environment

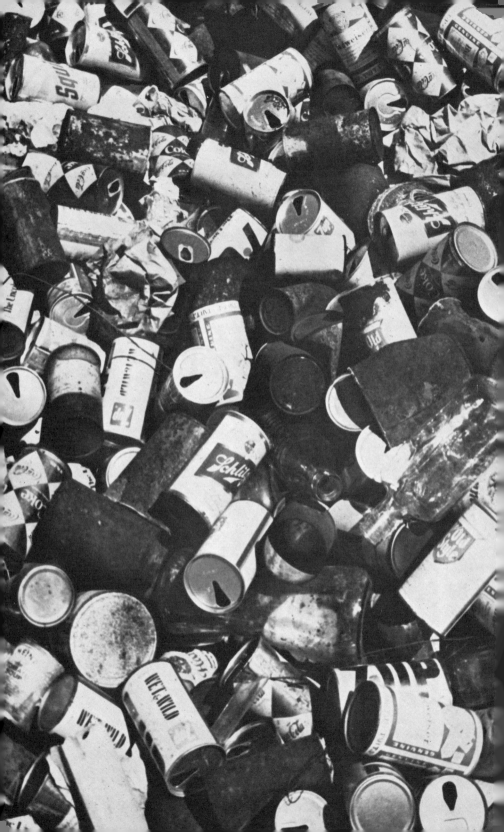

Man
Health and
Environment

Edited by

Brent Q. Hafen
Department of Health Science
Brigham Young University
Provo, Utah

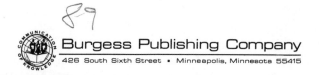
Burgess Publishing Company
426 South Sixth Street • Minneapolis, Minnesota 55415

1   2   3   4   5   6   7   8   9

Frontispiece photo courtesy of Henry H. Valiukas,
Minnesota Environmental Control Citizens Association (MECCA).

Preface

The following comments are indicative of our recent national concern for the health consequences of environmental pollution:

> Dire predictions of the health dangers from environmental contamination are routine in the news media and are common topics of daily conversation. Some of the allegations are sound; others patently alarmist and exaggerated, for many important data are lacking. In the last decade it has become clear that the problem is too urgent to be brushed lightly aside and that ignorance must be replaced with information.[1]

It is evident that the nature of our public health problems have changed over the years. Our past public health efforts to protect our communities from disease must be enlarged to include the provision for protection of our health against the increasing complexity of an expanding, changing, and highly complex technological society. It is this increase in technology, coupled with a deteriorating environment, that has resulted in a more detailed and serious consideration of the health implications of such pollution. It does seem that technological advances which have helped in the past to conquer

---

[1]*Man's Health and the Environment–Some Research Needs, a Report of Task Forces on Research and Planning in Environmental Health Sciences.* U.S. Department of Health, Education and Welfare, Public Health Services. National Institute of Environmental Health Sciences 1970.

many of our dreaded diseases have created many other health problems. These relate to air and water pollution, ionizing radiation, the stresses and strains of noise, speed, light, and congestion—as well as such things as chemical contamination, food processing, population growth, etc. It is apparent that we cannot continue in the same careless pattern if we are to protect our health and the environment. Even though great strides have been made in the past public health efforts, these are crucial times that require effort on everyone's part if we are to achieve a more esthetic and healthful environment. This requires that each of us in our own discipline and community (1) recognize the serious threat of environmental pollution; (2) be alerted to the various pollutants that have a detrimental affect on human health; and (3) develop programs within our disciplines and communities for preventing and controlling those health problems that may arise from environmental pollution.

The purpose of this book of readings is to provide an overview of the nature and effect of the various types of the environmental pollutants with particular emphasis on the latest available scientific knowledge of the health and welfare hazards of such pollution.

This compilation of readings should be of particular interest to anyone who is teaching in the area of the environmental sciences or any of the health-related subjects. These readings have been gathered from numerous sources and revolve around the following general areas:

A. Health and Environmental Pollution
B. Air Pollution
C. Water and Solid Wastes
D. Noise and Radiation
E. Toxic Substances
F. Population Growth
G. Environmental Education

An effort has been made to include readings on a variety of environmental health areas. However, it is important to realize that this collection is only a small sample of what is available in the literature; and it is intended to be only a general introduction to the problems surrounding environmental health.

Brent Q. Hafen

Provo, Utah
January, 1972

Contents

Introduction

During 1970, The World Health Organization intensified its studies on environmental health, giving greater prominence to human ecology. Work has started on a long-term program concerned with water, soil, food and air pollution as well as with noise and other environmental factors potentially harmful to human health.

Man relies on the dispersing, diluting and stabilizing capacities of air, water and soil to assimilate wastes and maintain the environmental balance necessary to support life. To the known pollutants such as the human wastes and air-borne particles and gases from the combustion of fuel are added discharges from industry. They are composed of a variety of residues of ever-increasing chemical complexity. Some wastes are returned to the natural cycle by the environmental self-purification process, others are not. Some pollutants, such as chlorinated hydrocarbon pesticides, mercury, and also some micro-organisms and radionucleids are incorporated in the food chain.

When waste products are discharged at a rate that overwhelms the natural forces of dispersion, dilution and decomposition, they can make the environment hazardous for human health. During the last few years the general public has become progressively aware of the dangers of pollution and the governments of both developed and developing countries are making efforts to establish monitoring systems, to enact basic legislation and to initiate national programs for pollution control.[1]

Even though there is often uncertainty as to what specific environmental changes do to human health, it is obvious that today's environment is having an adverse impact on the physical, emotional, and social health of increasing numbers of Americans.

[1]Excerpt from "Developing a Strategy," *World Health,* May, 1971.

I. UNDERSTANDING

ENVIRONMENTAL HEALTH

PROBLEMS

Pollution

Luther L. Terry

I cannot agree with the remark attributed to George Bernard Shaw, "Science is always wrong. It never solves a problem without creating ten more." On the other hand, I believe we have to face up to the challenge implicit in this remark—that is, we must reap the benefits of modern science and at the same time protect ourselves against the inherent possible hazards.

Today, we live in an increasingly mechanized, urbanized, man-made environment. The consequences are apparent on every hand. Science has formulated compounds and introduced techniques which have been seized upon by man eager to improve his daily living. And so we live with a vast complexity of man-made pollutants.

Our obligation is inescapable. It must be pointed out—emphatically, clearly, and repeatedly—that contamination of our environment poses dangers which science and society must solve together for their mutual benefit.

It is difficult to pinpoint the complex nature of the health danger from specific environmental pollutants. It is difficult to alert people to the importance of effects that are delayed in their nature and uncertain in their impact. But the message is one we must carry forward.

In devising the means to shape our world harmoniously, let's consider the value of an ecological approach to the environment. Ecology has been defined by Aldous Huxley as the science of the "mutual relations of organisms with their environment and with one another."

Man has often regarded certain specific geographical areas as simply a source of crops, minerals, wood products, or game for his own use. To release into an area a chemical product which has the purpose of destroying one form of life, without recognizing and taking into account the effects of this product on other forms of life, is short-sighted. The ecological approach suggests that these broad geographic areas be regarded not only as organic wholes but as related to others and alterable only with great caution.

The current interest in environmental health then embraces a positive interest in ecology. In any discussion of ecology and environmental health, we

Reprinted by permission from *Today's Education. NEA Journal.* January 1970.

hear a great deal about "adaptation"—man's ability or inability, to adjust to his environment and his genius, or foolhardiness, in seeking to adapt the environment to himself. I am suggesting that the greatest problem bearing upon environmental health in our time is another kind of adaptation—an adaptation in human thinking.

One does not have to be a chemist or a biologist to recognize that the interaction of several environmental stresses may produce an effect greater than the sum of their separate influences. We will not be able to comprehend the real place of man in his environment until we have assimilated the ecological concept into our thinking. As we reexamine our philosophy, we must also readjust our scientific, social, and economic goals to reflect an appreciation of these implications. Ecological wisdom must become a part of scientific thought and a force in social and economic behavior.

A splintering of programs and research has caused the environmental health effort to resemble, at times, Henry Adams' definition of philosophy, "unintelligible answers to insoluble problems." We are, however, making some progress toward a unified ecological view. As we do so, the problems do not appear insoluble. I believe that we are coming up with some intelligible answers.

Let us examine the various aspects of environmental pollution, air pollution, water pollution, occupational health hazards, radiological health hazards, and the need for environmental engineering and food protection. Even though I shall deal with them separately, I want to emphasize that they are separate facets of the same problem. The same chemicals may impinge on the individual in air, in milk, in foods, in water, and in his occupational environment—not once but repeatedly. Analysis of the parts, however, is still essential to an understanding of the whole.

Air pollution is, of course, a problem created primarily by urbanization. But air pollution is not limited to large centers of population. Even by 1960, it was estimated that over 300 urban communities in the United States had major air pollution problems, and 850 communities, moderate problems. The number of communities having minor but still recognizable air pollution problems, however, ran into several thousand. Only within the last 15 years has science begun to gather precise knowledge of the nature, extent, and effects of air pollution. We have learned that the air is charged with a multitude of particulate and gaseous pollutants whose adverse effects are both more subtle and more extensive than was once assumed.

Research has demonstrated that a link exists between air pollution and such major respiratory diseases as asthma, bronchitis, emphysema, cancer and possibly even the common cold. Even if no other basis existed, this would indicate that the nation's control of the pollutants ought to be greatly increased. But the deleterious effects of polluted air are not confined to the human respiratory system. Plants and animals are also adversely affected by air pollution. Agricultural losses, the destruction of property, and lowered real estate values are among the effects of air pollution that are costing this country many billions of dollars each year.

The federal government is fully committed to a course of action that is intended to result in better control of air pollution throughout the United States. Since 1955, when the Congress first enacted legislation dealing with air pollution, the responsibiltiy for federal air pollution activities has been assigned to the Department of Health, Education, and Welfare. Two units of the Public Health Service conducted the air pollution program until 1960, when the Division of Air Pollution was created. In 1967, the Division became the National Center for Air Pollution Control.

Progress toward control of air pollution depends upon an increasing fund of knowledge about its sources, nature, and effects. The Clean Air Act of 1963 recognized the need for this kind of information. The Act authorized expansion of the federal program of direct and supported research in a number of specific areas, among them automotive exhaust and the emissions associated with the use of sulfur-bearing coal and fuel oils.

In 1965, when it became apparent that national control of motor vehicle pollution was technically feasible, the Clean Air Act was amended to enable the Secretary of Health, Education, and Welfare to establish appropriate standards and to empower him to investigate and seek to prevent potential legal problems resulting from attempts to control air pollution problems. In 1966, the Act was further amended to authorize federal grants to state and local agencies to assist them in maintaining effective air pollution control programs; this supplemented already existing authority to promote the development, establishment, or improvement of such programs.

The strengthened national effort made possible by the Clean Air Act is a challenge to the scientific and engineering community. If man is to preserve and protect the air he breathes, we must continue to add to our knowledge of this problem and to apply the results of this knowledge promptly and effectively.

Because of pollution, our national water supply is threatened. Lakes and rivers have been befouled by deposits of municipal, industrial, and agricultural wastes. Beaches have had to be closed to swimming and fishing. Finding enough clean water for year-round municipal supply is touch-and-go in a number of areas. Many underground water resources are already in jeopardy.

The list of water pollutants is formidable. It includes plant nutrients that cause unpleasant tastes and odors and steal oxygen from our water supply; synthetic chemicals, dissolved minerals, and other substances from mining and industrial operations and from land drainage; as well as radioactive substances, heat from industrial processes, and soil sediments and mineral particles washed from the land by rain or floodwaters. The problems these pollutants present are so complex, so varied, and so numerous that existing weapons are not adequate to deal with them. They have multiplied faster than solutions.

The passage of the Water Quality Act of 1965 and of the Clean Water Restoration Act of 1966 marked the beginning of a major offensive against water pollution in this country. In response to this legislation, the Federal Water Pollution Control Administration of the Department of the Interior sponsors research that runs the gamut of scientific investigation and technological development—from basic research through applied research, pilot plants, field evaluation, and demonstration projects.

One basic long-range objective of the research is to be able to control waste at its source. The techniques range from abating acid mine drainage to encouraging changes in the construction of the waste processes of new industrial plants. Advanced waste treatment is one of the most dramatic examples of the full-scale demonstration of new treatment techniques. A breakthrough in this area will result in the development of effective, safe, and economical waste water systems which will, in effect, amount to the same thing as the creation of a new water supply.

Another old, but difficult water pollution problem confronts urban areas— the discharge of mixed raw sewage and storm water into our streams. To engineers of a previous era, it seemed logical to collect both storm water and sanitary sewage in a single combined system, since this provided marked savings. But these overflows are now recognized as carriers of pollutants into the watercourses.

The first Federal Water Pollution Control Act, passed in 1956, initiated a program of federal grants to municipalities to assist them in improving on building sewage treatment works. Amendments since then have helped to step up construction activity by making more money available on a more liberal basis.

The construction grants program has accomplished much since its beginning. In the first 12 years of the program, spurred by more than $1.4 billion in federal grants, some 9,500 treatment facilities, costing a total of $6.1 billion, were constructed or expanded.

Impressive as it has been, progress has not kept pace with needs. To deal with the large quantities of untreated or inadequately treated municipal wastes that still pour into waters across the country, municipalities will have to build waste treatment works on a vaster scale than ever before.

Without any doubt, ecological sensitivity appears almost mandatory if we are to succeed in solving the multitude of problems related to our most crucial national resource—water. The various interests of the wildlife conservationist, the fisherman, the farmer, and the guardian of human health find a common purpose in maintaining the purity and abundance of an untainted water supply.

Rivers die silently. Pollution robs us of clean water sometimes before we are aware of what is happening. One of the difficulties in combating water pollution is that the enemy is so often invisible. Even our most advanced analytical procedures have difficulty in detecting the substances lurking in water. It is evident, I think, that a clear concept of proper water use must take into consideration forests, national parks, wildlife, industry, municipalities—almost every aspect of our environment, present and future.

The health problems of workers illustrate very aptly, I think, the interrelatedness of all environmental hazards. The worker is the first to be exposed to most of the chemical and physical hazards which later pose a threat to the general population. In addition, there is a growing indication that occupation may directly contribute to the incidence of various chronic or deteriorating diseases previously believed to be entirely unconnected with work exposure.

Because fewer than 15 million of the 53 million wage and salary workers in industries are provided in-plant health service, identification of occupationally related disease is often difficult, and mechanisms for reporting their incidence and prevalence are inadequate.

In the meantime, technological changes bring new and exotic threats to worker health—from the insidious wastes of liquid oxygen fuel to the lasers and plasma torches that are finding increased application in industry. Some strains in the occupational climate have definite bearing on mental and emotional health. Pressing for attention, for example, are the health implications of noise, speed, work pressures, crowding, and others.

In this age of technology, close scrutiny of occupation exposures and development of worker protection are among the first requirements for maintaining a healthy environment.

The prevention of radiological health hazards is another one of the primary tasks confronting us. Among the things we do not know, are: (a) exactly how much radiation our population is being exposed to in the aggregate from various sources; (b) what the long-term effects of radiation are on man; and (c) how we can best protect ourselves from these effects.

We are continuing to monitor and to study whether there are any effects of fallout from testing nuclear devices. The limited test ban treaty of October 1963 was not only a significant step toward world peace; it substantially reduced a major threat to health. We are now free to make a larger effort toward the control of other sources of radioactivity. Among these are nuclear reactors used for power and production, medical and industrial X rays, and microwave ovens and lasers. At the present time, the greatest man-made source is X ray, which is estimated to contribute about one-half of all ionizing radiation exposure to the general population.

One of our activities is off-site monitoring at missile test sites. Our Radiation Alert Network of 74 stations throughout the nation serves as an early alert system by monitoring gross beta radioactivity in air. We also collect milk samples at 63 stations in all parts of the country for radionuclide analysis and estimate the total dietary intake of radionuclides in an institutional diet sampling now being carried on in every state.

There is no doubt that public health activity relating to radiation exposure of the public will continue to grow with increased application of electronic devices capable of emitting ionizing as well as nonionizing radiation, the use of radioisotopes, medical and dental X rays, and nuclear power reactors. Reduction and control of exposure will require a concerted effort in research, surveillance, and training, as well as in application and enforcement of the Radiation Control for Health and Safety Act of 1968.

The interrelationship between all these aspects of environmental health is complex. No less complicated is the relationship existing in public administration relating to environmental health. The difficulties encountered in developing urban sanitary facilities, for example, are not necessarily due to technical problems, nor even to financial obstacles. In many instances, failures may be traced to jurisdictional tangles, to gaps or overlaps or conflicts in environmental health responsibility.

The Public Health Service's Division of Environmental Engineering and Food Protection directly assists communities seeking practical, ecologically sound solutions to these problems.

Insects and rodents, for example, are no respecters of county lines. Furthermore, the recent outbreaks of mosquito-borne encephalitis show that existing measures are not always adequate to prevent disease.

In our sprawling and expanding metropolitan areas, urban planning cannot begin and end at the city boundary. Without coordinated planning, we will invade more farmland and bulldoze more forests to make room for housing developments, shopping centers, and industries. Sewage and refuse will be handled in whatever way seems easiest and cheapest at the moment.

Even our park areas—today visited by a growing number of people— compound the environmental health problem. Water supply, food protection, and waste disposal in parks and campgrounds affect thousands of tourists. And every year, more and more people are exposed to encephalitis, Rocky Mountain spotted fever, tick fever, and tularemia.

The revolution in food technology in the last few years has been a radical one. A variety of precooked frozen foods are available for our convenience. New methods of processing and merchandising foods have been introduced. Additives and preservatives may have unsuspected health effects. In spite of tremendous advances in food handling, there are still over one million cases each year of illness due to the ingestion of contaminated foods.

In all these areas—primarily related to environmental engineering and sanitation—the Public Health Service is charged with providing coordination and national leadership. It also has certain direct federal responsibilities for the inspection and enforcement of sanitation regulations in interstate commerce. Its Division of Environmental Engineering and Food Protection assists in long-range environmental health planning; prepares sanitation standards for milk, food, shellfish and food services; and provides consultation on individual water supply, sewage disposal, and other health problems.

Private scientific institutions have turned their attention to the environmental sciences and are making their own substantial contributions to the total fund of knowledge. Obviously, different techniques may be required to cope with the threats present in different sectors of the environment. But we regard the man-environment relationship as being "one and indivisible."

It is quite clear, I think, that maintaining a healthful environment today requires the coordinated effort of all levels of government, and all areas of science.

It has been said that the philosophies of one age become the absurdities of the next; and that the foolishness of yesterday becomes the wisdom of tomorrow. In the area of environmental health, tomorrow is already at hand—and fortunately we are beginning to acquire the wisdom to cope with some of the many complexities involved.

Human Ecology

Rene Dubos

Nowadays there is a tendency to believe that modern medicine consists exclusively of a few sensational recent discoveries—miracle drugs, spectacular techniques, sophisticated immunization methods. This tendency is dangerous, for it deflects attention from another aspect of modern medicine which is just as remarkable and perhaps of greater practical importance. If the health of the public has improved in many regions during recent decades, the improvement is due not only to certain specialized medical procedures, but also—and probably to a greater extent—to a better understanding of the effects of man's environment and way of life on his physiological and mental state. Our health is better than that of our ancestors to the extent that our lives are more in accord with what I would choose to call biological wisdom. The scientific expression of that biological wisdom is human ecology, i.e., knowledge of the relationships between man and the innumerable factors of his environment.

It would be easy and pleasant for me to devote this entire lecture to an inventory of the progress of modern medical science. But I feel that it will be more productive to consider in what respects that science is inadequate, particularly when it comes to coping with the new ecological crisis that at the present time is threatening almost every country in the world.

The word "environment" has in our day acquired an ever more tragic connotation, both in primitive agrarian societies and in industrial urban societies. It connotes, for example, malnutrition and infection in most of the poor countries, chemical pollution and mechanization of life in all the prosperous countries. The ecological crisis is everywhere so menacing and takes such varied forms that the term "human ecology" has come to be used only for certain situations that might lead to biological or mental disaster. Yet human ecology embraces far more than this tragic view of the relationships between man and his environment. Ecology teaches us that all the physical, biological, and social forces acting upon man impart a direction to his development and thus mold his nature. The body and the mind are constantly being modified, and hence shaped, by the stimuli that induce formative reactions. It is to be hoped that a

Reprinted by permission from *WHO Chronicle,* World Health Organization. Volume 23, No. 11.

time will come when human ecology will be able to pay greater attention to the positive and beneficial effects of the environment than to its pathogenic effects.

The social mechanisms whereby society tries to create a more or less artificial environment better adapted to man's needs and desires constitute an extremely important aspect of human ecology which I shall not attempt to discuss here. The other aspect of human ecology consists of the biological processes whereby the organism as a whole tries to adapt itself to environmental forces. The importance of these adaptive phenomena for health has frequently been demonstrated in the course of history. I shall mention a few examples of this.

In the narrative of his travels, Christopher Columbus speaks with admiration of the magnificent physical condition of the natives he discovered in Central America. In the eighteenth century, Cook, Bougainville, and the other navigators who ranged over the Pacific also wondered at the excellent health of the island population of Oceania. Many other explorers were similarly impressed on their first contact with the Indians, the Africans, and later, the Eskimos. The legend of the noble savage, healthy and happy, thus has its origin in the descriptions published by the explorers who observed certain native populations when they were still undeveloped and almost completely isolated from the rest of the world.

There was certainly a lot of false romanticism in the illusion that the noble savage was free from disease and social restrictions because he lived in a state of nature. But, all the same, this romantic and over-simplified view of man's estate has been partly justified by the studies in physical and social anthropology conducted on what contemporary anthropologists call man the hunter. These studies were recently the subject of a symposium under that title, in the course of which descriptions were given of the characteristics of populations that live without agriculture and even without tools, except for a few primitive objects they employ to derive their sustenance from wild plants and animals. It appears that this way of life, though so close to nature and therefore lacking any medical assistance, is compatible with a good state of health. But I like to emphasize the fact that primitive populations undergo rapid physical and mental deterioration as soon as they come into close contact with the modern world, and thus lose their ancestral manners and customs. The noble savage who seemed so healthy and happy in the eighteenth century had often become a human wreck by the nineteenth.

The epidemiological facts suggest that the good health of primitive peoples, like that of wild animals, is a manifestation of a biological equilibrium between the living creature and its environment. This equilibrium persists as long as the conditions of human ecology remain stable, but is broken as soon as the conditions change. The enormous problems of malnutrition, alcoholism, and infectious disease, which caused such a rapid physical deterioration among the primitive populations in the seventeenth, eighteenth, and nineteenth centuries, recurred in all the Western countries at the outset of the Industrial Revolution, when their working classes, originating largely from agricultural regions, underwent massive and sudden exposure to conditions of life that were then new to them.

NO TIME FOR ADAPTION

Adaption to industrial society is now far advanced in the prosperous countries, but this is only a temporary phase. New problems are arising from the fact that the second Industrial Revolution is causing sudden and far-reaching changes in the physical environment and in everyday living, thus creating a new and as yet unstable ecological situation. The changes naturally bring their own specific dangers, which undoubtedly underlie what we nowadays call the diseases of civilization.

Indeed, we might say that in our day, human ecology is undergoing an almost universal crisis because man is not yet adapted, and probably never will become adapted, either to the biological impoverishment of the very poor countries or to certain environmental influences that the second Industrial Revolution has introduced into the rich countries. It might be supposed that man, since he still has the same genetic make-up as in the past, could once again use the biological mechanisms that enabled him in the Stone Age to colonize a large part of the globe, and so could adapt himself to the conditions of physiological impoverishment or industrial intoxication of present-day life. But this is neither certain nor even probable, because the present changes are of a kind almost without precedent in human history.

Until now, changes in the pattern of living have generally been so slow that it took several generations before they affected all classes of society. This slowness enabled the entire range of adaptive forces to be brought into play: physiological and even anatomical characteristics, as well as mental reactions and particularly social organization, little by little changed. Nowadays, on the contrary, everything changes so quickly that the processes of biological and social adaptation do not have time to come into play. Whether from the biological or the social point of view, the father's experience is now of practically no value to the son.

It is also a known fact that the human faculty of adaptation, great as it is, is not unlimited. It is quite possible that the stresses of present-day living are taking it near its extreme limits.

In the course of his evolution, man has constantly been exposed to inclement weather, fatigue, periodic famine, and infection. To survive these dangers, he has had to develop in his genetic code hereditary mechanisms that have facilitated certain processes of adaptation. But man now has to face dangers of another kind, without any precedent in the biological past of the human species. He probably does not possess adaptive mechanisms for all the new situations to which he is exposed. Moreover, the evolution of biological mechanisms is far too slow to keep up with the accelerated pace of technological and social change in the modern world.

It is certain, for example, that there is no possible means of adaptation to nutritional deficiencies that persist for long periods. Many children in their growth phase succumb to them. If they survive, they cannot satisfactorily realize the potentialities of their genetic endowment; they are condemned for the rest of their lives to anatomical, physiological, and mental atrophy. A population continuously subjected to nutritional deficiency can only degenerate.

Industrial technology has introduced into modern life a range of substances and situations that man has never known in his biological past. It is probable that he will never be able to adapt himself to the toxic effects of chemical pollution and of certain synthetic products; to the physiological and mental difficulties caused by lack of physical effort; to the mechanization of life; and to the presence of a wide variety of artificial stimulants. We should probably add to this list the disturbances to natural body rhythms arising from the almost complete divorce of modern life from cosmic cycles.

There are no grounds for the fear that all deviations from the natural order that result from technological change will be dangerous to health. Far from it. It remains true, however, that the more a population is exposed to modern technology the more it appears to be subject to certain forms of chronic and degenerative disease—conditions called for precisely that reason the diseases of civilization. Premature death caused by these diseases is not due to the lack of medical care. In the USA, for example, scientists and especially physicians have, paradoxically, a shorter life expectancy than other groups, although they belong to an economically privileged class. Certain demographic studies show that the life expectancy beyond the age of 35 may have decreased somewhat during the last few years in the big cities of the USA.

MAN'S AMAZING TOLERANCE

Everyday life seems to give the lie to the anxieties expressed in the previous pages, since modern man appears to be just as adaptable as Stone Age man. An extraordinary number of people have survived the terrible ordeals of modern war and the concentration camps. Throughout the world it is the most crowded and polluted cities, those in which life is at its most ruthless, that attract most people and it is their population that is increasing at the greatest rate. Men and women are working all the time in the middle of the infernal noise of machines and telephones, in an atmosphere polluted with chemical fumes and tobacco smoke.

This remarkable tolerance of man toward conditions so different from those in which he has evolved has given rise to the myth that, through technological and social progress he can modify his way of life and his environment indefinitely and without risk. That is simply not true. As stated earlier, modern man can only adapt himself insofar as the mechanisms of adaptation are potentially present in his genetic code. Furthermore, it is certain that in many cases the apparent ease with which man adapts himself biologically, socially, and culturally to new or unfavorable conditions constitutes, paradoxically, a threat to individual well-being and even to the future of the human race.

This paradox arises from the fact that the word "adaptation" cannot be applied unreservedly to the adjustments that enable human beings to survive and function under modern conditions. Indeed, in man, sociocultural forces distort the effects of the kind of adaptive mechanisms that operate in the animal kingdom.

For the biologists, the expression "Darwinian adaptation" implies harmony between a species and a given environment, a harmony that enables it to multiply and, at the appropriate moment, to invade new territory. In the terms of this definition, man would appear to be remarkably well adapted to the conditions of life that exist both in highly industrialized societies and in developing countries, since the world's population is continuing to increase and to occupy an ever greater proportion of the land surface of the globe. However, what would constitute a biological success for another species is a serious social threat to the human species. The dangers arising from the increase in world population show clearly that the Darwinian concept of adaptation cannot be used if the well-being of humanity is taken as a criterion of its biological success.

For the physiologist, a reaction to environmental stress is adaptive when it neutralizes the disturbing effects of such stress on the body and mind. In general, physiological and psychological adaptive responses are a factor tending towards the well-being of the organism at the time when they occur. In man, however, they may in the long term have detrimental effects. Man is capable of acquiring some degree of tolerance toward environmental pollution, excessive stimuli, a harrassing social life in a competitive atmosphere, a rhythm completely foreign to natural biological cycles, and all the other consequences of his living in the world of cities and technology. This tolerance enables him to resist successfully exposure to influences which, at the outset, are unpleasant or traumatic. However, in many cases such tolerance is only acquired through a set of organic and mental processes that risk giving rise to degenerative manifestations.

THE THREAT OF IMPOVERISHED HUMANITY

Man can also learn to put up with the ugliness of the environment in which he lives, with its smoky skies and polluted streams. He can live without the scent of flowers, the song of birds, the life-enhancing spectacle of nature, and the other biological stimuli of the physical world. The suppression of a number of the pleasurable aspects of life and the stimuli that have conditioned his biological and mental evolution may have no manifest deleterious effect on his physical appearance or on his efficiency as a cog in the economic or technological machine, but there is a risk that, in the long run, it may impoverish his life and lead to the gradual loss of the qualities we associate with the idea of a human being.

Air, water, soil, fire, and the natural rhythms and diversity of living species are important not only as chemical combinations, physical forces, or biological phenomena but also because it is under their influence that human life has been fashioned. They have created in man deep-rooted needs that will not change in any near future. The pathetic weekend exodus toward the countryside or the beaches, the fireplaces that are still built in overheated urban apartments, the sentimental attachments formed for animals or even plants all bear witness to the survival deep down in man of biological and emotional urges acquired in the course of his evolution, of which he cannot rid himself.

Like the giant Antaeus in the Greek legend, man loses his strength as soon as he loses contact with the earth.

Human ecology therefore requires a scientific and intellectual attitude differing from that which would be adequate in general biology and even in the other biomedical sciences, because it has to deal with the indirect and long term effects exercised by the environment and way of life, even if those factors have no apparent immediate influence. It would be easy to illustrate the importance of those indirect and long-term effects by discussing, for example, the part played by the abundance or scarcity of food, the various forms of chemical and microbial pollution, the effects of noise or other stimuli, the density of and especially the rapid changes in the population; in brief, all of the environmental forces that act on man in every social class and in every country. Here, however, I shall confine myself to pointing out that the most important effects of the environment and way of life are often difficult to recognize because they only show themselves indirectly and after a lapse of time.

The early stages of life are of exceptional importance because to a large extent they determine what the adult will become. The young organism never forgets anything. All the factors that act upon it therefore contribute to the psychosomatic formation of the individual. The younger the person, the more malleable he is and the more easily affected by environmental influences. Hence the importance of the first stages of life, including those within the womb. These long-term and indirect manifestations of the environment are still poorly understood, but it is fortunately possible and even easy to study them experimentally since in animals, as in man, prenata conditions have a profound and often irreversible effect, bearing on the anatomical features of the adult as well as on metabolism and behavior. Animal experiments will therefore make it possible to see what is not easily seen in man, to understand what is not obvious to our minds and, consequently, to take action with a view to alleviating certain untoward or even disastrous consequences of the influences to which man is exposed at the beginning of his life.

Of course the environment continues unceasingly to transform the organism. However, the first years of life have effects so profound and irreversible that they are the most important part of human ecology. I am emphasizing this fact because it seems to me that it should influence the general policy of WHO and encourage scientists to devote more effort to the problems of childhood. It is beyond doubt that the establishment of an atmosphere favorable to the biological and mental development of the child is the most economical way of improving world health.

A better understanding of the effect of environment at the beginning of life on growth and development gives a deeper sense to the definition of health made famous by the preamble to the WHO Constitution: "Health is a state of complete physical, mental and social well-being and not merely an absence of disease or infirmity." This "positive health" advocated by WHO implies that a person should be able to express as completely as possible the potentialities of his genetic heritage. That heritage, however, can only find true expression to the extent that the environment transforms genetic potentialities into phenotypic realities. It is in this way that human ecology might finally become identified, as I expressed the hope that it could at the beginning of this lecture, with the positive and beneficial effects of the environment.

The word "health" in the sense that I have chosen to give it describes not a state but a potentiality—the ability of an individual or a social group to modify himself or itself continually not only in order to function better in the present but also to prepare for the future. Ideal health will, however, always remain a mirage, because everything in our life will continue to change. The doctor and the public health expert are in the same position as the gardener or farmer faced with insects, molds, and weeds. Their work is never done. Man quickly grows tired of conditions of life that had originally seemed attractive. Individually and collectively he will look for adventure, and this forces him to live under constantly new conditions, with all the unforeseen occurrences and threats to health involved in change.

There is no question, however, of turning back. A society that does not move forward quickly deteriorates. Indeed, it cannot even survive in a world where everything is in a state of flux. Civilizations can only succeed and survive by exploring the unknown and accepting the risks involved in plunging ahead into the future. Technology would soon cease to develop if a certificate of absolute safety were required for every technical innovation and every new product.

It is therefore inevitable that economic and social progress should always be accompanied by hazards to health whatever the advances made by medicine and hygiene.

This fact gives the doctor and the hygienist a still more important social role than they have at the present moment. It consists in recognizing as swiftly as possible, and even in anticipating, the medical problems that will arise increasingly as a result of the accelerated rate of technological and economic innovation. For this purpose it is becoming urgent to set up what might be called listening posts to record the first signs of pathological disorders that might threaten to spread to society as a whole. For example, the effects of atmospheric pollution, changes in food habits, the almost universal and constant use of new drugs, and automation in industry and in every aspect of life are still unforeseeable but could doubtless be detected before health disasters become widespread. It is a matter of satisfaction that this social responsibility is already recognized in certain sectors of the public service. Thus thorough studies of the biological effects of ionizing radiation have been undertaken with a view to developing in advance practical methods of protection against the probable consequences of the industrial use of radiation. There would be no point in quoting here studies of the same kind already undertaken by WHO on the effect of drugs and insecticides. This farsighted attitude will have to be generally adopted. In the future the development of technological innovations should always include parallel scientific studies on the long-term effects of these innovations on human ecology.

As Jacques Parisot wrote, "To cure is good but to prevent is better." Humanity will only be able to avoid the hazards of the future by extending its scientific knowledge and showing greater social conscience.

Environmental Health and Mental Health

Eric W. Mood
Morris Shiffman
Dorothea C. Leighton

INTRODUCTION

During the past two decades there have been vast changes in the field of public health, not least in the areas subsumed by environmental health. These changes have been a response to the exigencies brought about by: (1) a rapid increase in population; (2) a precipitous expansion of the industrial economy; (3) applications of scientific discoveries leading to the development of new materials, products and services; (4) mobility of the population, plus its concentration in urban areas; (5) a profound realignment of social, economic, and cultural values; (6) a general improvement in living standards; and (7) an increase in available leisure time. Singly and in combination, these developments and trends have had important impact on man's biological, chemical, physical, and social environments.

In an attempt to find solutions to some of these problems, government and society have addressed themselves to aspects of many issues, but generally along traditional lines; e.g., solutions to problems of chemical pollution have been sought within the chemical environment. A number of governmental reports of the past decade reflect an attempt to define problems of environmental pollution and to recommend possible solutions (1-10).

A philosophy of public health was expressed in 1960 by Dr. Leroy E. Burney, then Surgeon General, U.S. Public Health Service, who said:

> The health status of an individual, a community or a nation is determined by the interplay and integration of two ecological universes: the internal environment of man himself; the external environment of the world as it affects him. . . . In considering the external environment, three major areas of health concern are recognized:
> 1. The biological component, including the living things of the plant and animal kingdoms—ranging from the food upon which life depends to those micro-organisms responsible for disease.

Reprinted from *Mental Health Considerations In Public Health,* Health Services and Mental Health Administration, National Institute of Mental Health, Public Health Services Publication # 1898, May 1969.

2. The physical component, encompassing the nonliving things and physical forces affecting man—such as water, air, food, chemicals, heat, light, and other radiations.

3. The social component, including a complex interplay of factors and conditions—cultural values, customs, attitudes, and mores; economic status, social and political organizations, and ability to support facilities and services.

These components are closely interrelated (11).

This philosophy of public health has not been accepted completely by public health workers as they have sought to achieve a higher level of health for everyone. The failure to understand the interplay and required integration of the two ecological universes, or to take account of the biological, physical, and social areas of health concern that are inevitable parts of man's external environment, may explain why definitions of current health problems tend to lack comprehensiveness, and why recommended solutions provide but palliative remedies at best.

Setting the limits of the term "environmental health" as it will be used in the material to follow is particularly pressing since many meanings have been associated with these words. Some definitions, such as the one used by the Task Force on Environmental Health, National Commission on Community Health Services, are too limiting because the social aspects have been omitted (12).

A more satisfactory definition was proposed by the Ad Hoc Committee on Training in Environmental Health which, in 1960, submitted its report to the Association of Schools of Public Health. Its definition states that "environmental health deals with the impact of the physical, biological, and social environment of man and with the adjustments and controls of external factors to promote his health and well-being" (13). This definition specifically includes the social as well as the physical and biological aspects of environment, and involves the interactions of man with the various elements of his environment, including their adjustments and controls. We will adopt this definition for present purposes.

For the purposes of this paper, "environmental health" as used herewith will exclude the occupational environment, a subject which should be discussed in any comprehensive statement of environmental health.

Environmental health thus defined is not seen as the sole province of any one group or level of professionals. Rather, the definition is meant to apply to all persons whose activities fall within the stated scope, whether engineer or nonengineer, physician or nonphysician, and whatever the level of academic training.

DEFINITION OF MENTAL HEALTH

The abstract nature of the phenomenon labeled "mental health," plus the tendency to use the term also to mean "mental illness," point to the need for a fairly full statement of the concept that will be employed in this paper. Thinking of it, then, as a state which has a range from positive to negative, what can be said about it? The first point is that one's state of mental health is roughly synonymous with one's state of adaptation—adequate or inadequate. Secondly, it includes components which are affected by everything that goes on in its environment, whether physical, social, or psychological. Finally, if not understood and taken into account, it can thwart the best conceived plan for environmental improvement by its negative aspects. It thus becomes an environmental factor which an environmental scientist should comprehend and respect.

The degree to which the mental (or adaptive) state is healthy or unhealthy depends upon the dynamic balance of the moment between the various internal and external systems which determine the ability of the person to cope, on the one hand, and give him something to cope with, on the other. Internal systems are determined in part by heredity, in part by life experience and by the patterns established, to date, by coping behavior. A stabilized external situation makes it possible for a comparatively stable personal-environmental equilibrium to develop.

Disturbances, however, can be initiated either within or outside the person. A thought, a feeling, or a perception can trigger a series of physiological changes and voluntary or involuntary reactions which may lead to some kind of observable action or to internally felt pleasure or pain. Noise or silence, light or darkness, crowding or isolation, as examples of a myriad of external changes, may lead to the same (or to a different) chain of reactions, according to the way in which a person's previous experience leads him to interpret the particular external condition.

To progress a little beyond the simple stimulus-response level, some of the social aspects of man's existence will be examined. Related to the helpless condition in which the human infant is born, he must become a social animal, cared for by others until able to care for himself. Families were probably formed because it was an advantage to each parent to have the other one perform part of the work involved in rearing their young. Families clustered together for similar reasons, and today an enormous huddle of families in the cities is found, due in large part to industrialization and mechanization which has caused people to leave farming areas and to seek work where factories are concentrated in order to find support for themselves.

Social scientists (preceded by philosophers) have given much thought to specifying basic human needs for adequate adaptation, and have produced a number of lists. Although the lists vary in some details, there is considerable overlap. A summary of the needs discussed in one source (14) runs as follows:

I. *Biological-environmental:*
   a. Physical security (food, shelter, health); and
   b. Sexual satisfaction.

II. *Psychological-environmental:*
  a. Opportunity to express hostility without reprisal;
  b. Opportunity to express and secure love;
  c. Opportunity to secure recognition;
  d. Opportunity to express spontaneity, creativity, volition, etc.; and
  e. Basic "esthetic satisfaction."

III. *Social-environmental:*
  a. Orientation in terms of one's place in society and the places of others;
  b. Securing and maintaining membership in a definite human group; and
  c. Sense of belonging to a moral order (a system of values) and of being right in what one does.

The assumption is that man exists in a state of striving for these items, and that interference with his achieving them constitutes a strain on his adaptational ability which may result in the development of symptoms that may eventually reach the proportions of mental illness. Research and experience confirm that many people get along well with fairly marked interferences with some items on the list, and that the absence of any one item is hardly ever crucial (with the exception, of course, of a minimal amount of food). On the whole, however, good mental health (adequate adaptation) is most often associated with a satisfactory amount of most of the items, and poor mental health (inadequate adaptation) is usually associated with multiple lacks (15).

In stable societies, large or small, arrangements develop to provide for the kinds of needs listed. Physical security, for example, requires the development of ways of providing food, such as agriculture, food preservation, distribution systems, and some means of exchange so that agricultural products can be paid for in other goods, services, or money. It further requires housing and clothing, which imply architectural styles and heating for the housing, and the development of fabrics and means of fitting them to the human form for the clothing. Health demands a source of water, safe disposition of excrement and other wastes, and a means of dealing with illness which often stimulates the development of medico-religious specialists. Sexual satisfaction basically requires a sufficient number of persons of both sexes and appropriate ages, but usually is also an activity that is subject to social regulation which specifies, at least, the degree of relationship between individuals who engage in legitimate sex activity.

All the other needs listed are predicated upon some sort of human grouping which, over time and through interaction among its members and with its bio-physico-chemical environment, develops patterns of behavior and institutions which will provide reasonably adequate adaptation for the majority of its members.

When marked social, cultural, or environmental change takes place, however, a long period of time may elapse before a new and satisfactory equilibrium can be established, and a great deal of personal and societal disequilibrium may result which throws many people into an inadequate state of adaptation (or mental "illth"). The loss of stability may affect members of the society at different times and in various ways, according to the original organization of the group and the kind of change that occurs. A contemporary example of this sort of change is the industrialization-urbanization now so widespread in the world. The drastic personal upset attendant upon giving up an open, rural, agricultural existence (which depends to a large extent upon the seasonal and diurnal rhythms of nature) for the clock-bound, crowded, unfamiliar life of the city has well-documented repercussions in heightened blood pressure (16) for example, and in a rise of symptoms commonly associated with psychological stress (17).

Quite obviously, everything on the list, whether characterized as biological-, psychological-, or social-environmental, may or must involve social interactions. This perhaps underlines the importance of people to one another in both the positive and the negative sense, and the essentially social nature of departures from mental health (adequate adaptation) which will result from serious upsets in societal equilibrium. Such departures may appear in a variety of forms, ranging from psychophysiological symptoms, anxiety or depression, at one extreme, to psychotic manifestations at the other, in the most affected groups. Or it may show as aggressive acts against other persons, such as assault or child abuse.

As the preceding paragraph indicates, just as in the case of physical health, the way in which the level of mental health or adaptation is determined depends usually upon evaluating the level and types of symptoms indicating maladaptation of a group—if there is nothing detectable wrong with a group of people, they must be healthy. It is much more difficult to search out the balance of satisfaction or deprivation of the basic needs which have been discussed than it is to recognize and count the various symptoms and behaviors which signalize a breakdown in the balance. It is by some such symptom count that it is possible to understand better the interplay of environmental and human factors in a given situation, for one will find reflections in human behavior of deficits in basic needs due to environmental causes, including the contributions of the physical, chemical, and social factors to such lacks.

In summary, then, mental health is defined as a state of adequate adaptation to the biological-chemical-physical and social-psychological environment in which the person resides. On the whole, the term "mental health" leads to more misunderstanding than the term "adaptation." To the extent possible, "adaptation" will be used in this paper in lieu of "mental health."

ENVIRONMENT AND HUMAN REACTION

The enlargement of the professional's view as to the scope, content, and objectives of the field of environmental health has not drastically changed the established range of activities in the field. Even the introduction of new words such as "environmental quality" to describe the increased conceptual breadth of the field has not been reflected into new images. Gaffney (18) notes that the term "environmental quality" is loosely used by persons who actually are speaking about their own particular piece of the environmental pie. He says that "the environment of the slum dweller consists largely of houses and streets, joints and cheap stores, playgrounds and schools, garbage cans, and vibrations from neighborhood drop-forges." These are some of the urban environmental problems that are real, but not exciting to the professional. The professional is more concerned with the engineering, epidemiological, and toxicological considerations stemming from his professional orientation. This concept of environmental quality can be labeled better as pollution control and esthetic uplift from the viewpoint of the upper middle classes.

Environmentalists, however, are being urged by the public and legislators to direct their attention to the esthetic, social, and ethical aspects of man's use of his environment. They are further being directed to clarify their objectives for environmental change and to indicate the criteria by which these objectives will be satisfied in terms of social as well as economic and physical indicators. There are available indicators for the quantitative aspects of environmental pollution (both physical and economic). Qualitative indicators reflecting social benefit and livability are more difficult to formulate.

Fisher (19) deals with some of the problems of measurement of environmental quality and notes that these indicators are difficult to formulate because:

a. attitudes differ sharply as to what constitutes environmental quality;
b. there are conflicting objectives in the use of the environment; and
c. questions arise as to place and point in time where environmental quality shall be measured.

Social attitude and preference indicators are necessary to provide a more realistic criterion on which to base programs. For instance, food programs are based now on criteria of consumer acceptance, and on social preferences to a greater extent than on objectives emphasizing prevention of food-borne disease. These social indicators for a food protection program should be stated as explicitly as possible so that the public knows what they are getting, so that legislators know what the appropriations are for, and so that administrators should know what they are actually accomplishing towards achieving social goals. The same case may be made for air pollution control.

Minimum standards of air quality could be set in terms of selected physical characteristics, but the people should be allowed to choose to have more than these minimum standards. The people in the air-shed involved would have to find appropriate and democratic ways for reaching decisions about levels of air quality that would be desirable and practical from an economic and political point of view.

Fisher notes, "This information-gathering, discussion and decision process becomes of central importance . . . to the establishment of goals and standards. It is through processes of this sort that communities can move from the basic physical indicators to a consideration of social consequences and possibilities. The process requires a measurement of public attitude to environmental pollution, including considerations of mental health and well-being."

One may still ask the question, "Why is it important to assess public opinion on environmental pollution?" Lowenthal (18) has given the following reasons:

a. to give people an actual role in making decisions about their environment;

b. to smooth the path for making an executive decision. The decision maker makes himself aware of the client's preferences in advance and thereby can propose a course of action which is acceptable and capable of implementation;

c. finally, to alter public opinion. People may not be aware of the issues. Opinion polling may offer the public a chance to inform themselves of and to concern themselves with a problem.

How, then, do attitudes enter into decisionmaking? White (18) indicates that the process of attitude formation is not well-known at present, but we can assume that attitudes enter into a decision about environment in these ways:

a. through the personal attitudes of those people sharing in the decision-making which are directly expressed in the decision;

b. through one person's opinion as to what others prefer—and decisions are made in deference to such opinions; and,

c. there are the opinions of one group as to what others *should* prefer.

The latter opinion (c) may be the most influential factor in shaping attitudes on the modification of environmental pollution. These opinions derive from already formed attitudes of the administrator or the technical specialist which he attempts to impose on the community.

What is actually meant by attitude? White notes that the term "attitude" is used interchangeably with "belief" or "opinion" to describe a preference held by a person with respect to an object or a concept. It does not in itself constitute a value or mark of value; it is the result of a valuation process of some kind, and always involves a preference. Insofar as it applies to an aspect of the environment, it requires perception of that environment. A critical point with regard to perception is that it is always organized on the basis of a person's social experience. The same environmental condition (e.g., a stream or a backyard) may be perceived differently by two people. To one, the stream may be just an open drain, while to the other, it is a little bit of nature nostalgic of his childhood. Therefore, there are no absolute standards of esthetic experience, only standards which vary with **experience** and personality. Yet, in the well-recognized branch of environmental control dealing with public nuisances, there is an assumption of agreement among persons in their perception of what constitutes a nuisance. In fact, programs are organized, regulations written, and legal proceedings instituted on the premise that there is common agreement on what constitutes a detrimental environmental condition.

There is current interest in the application of attitude surveys to develop a better basis for standards for crowding, congestion, noise, odor, and general stress. The report, "A Strategy for a Livable Environment" (10), notes that these conditions are insidious threats to man's physical, mental, and social well-being. Yet, there are few studies on which to base the control activity. Such studies can only be done through the search for factors which relate the influence of physical states to mental attitudes and perceptions.

How may these attitudes and preferences be measured? The simplest answer is to look at the way people behave in the face of a specific stress or to ask them their preferences in relation to some specific condition. The investigator can question people about their attitudes and also about any maladaptive symptoms they may have developed. Some studies that have been made include:

a. The Outdoor Recreation Resources Review Commission. This was the first public agency to attempt a canvass of consumer demand for the use of recreational environments (20).

b. The Public Health Service has carried out a number of studies on Community Perception of Air Quality (21) to measure the extent of annoyance with air pollution expressed by persons in a city.

c. A study of "Public Awareness and Concern with Air Pollution in St. Louis" (22), which investigated the decisionmaking influence of attitudes, concludes that measuring the public awareness and concern with air pollution is necessary to any assessment of the problem. Such an assessment is needed to form the basis for a realistic control program.

d. The report on a "Strategy for a Livable Environment" (10) extended similar recommendations to include the total environment and noted that there was a need to "determine what social pressures and factors most forcefully influence public attitudes (including indifference) toward environmental problems." The lack of such information compels a pollution control agency to operate somewhat in the dark. The report contains a recommendation that urban sociological research centers be established in major metropolitan areas to study environmental influences on social well-being. Further, the need for using such information to mobilize public understanding and support for the control of environmental health problems is emphasized.

Sociology of Complaints about Nuisances

The lowly nuisance complaint has not received the share of attention that it really merits. The few studies that have been made are by sociologists who have been concerned with how people perceive environmental hazards and how the socio-demographic characteristics of the respondents relate to the level of the perceived hazards of smog, air traffic, noise, etc. (23), and by geographers and psychologists concerned with man's response to the physical environment (24).

The concept of the "nuisance" has long been recognized in public health activities. From both a legal and practical view there is an accepted definition of a nuisance as a commonly identified annoyance to the citizen. The level of insult created by the nuisance is recognized as sufficient for imposing corrective actions without the need for demonstrating that the physical health of the individual is endangered. The mental health component of the insult is tacitly accepted. However, in practice there is a difficulty in deciding whether an annoyance or a basis for complaint really exists. This occurs because there are a number of personal factors operative in nuisance complaints. The expression of the nuisance complaint, therefore, becomes dependent on the interplay between:

a. the actual nature of the environmental stress; and

b. the characteristics of the individual and his motivation for complaining.

The same level of stress will be perceived differently by different individuals. Sociologists have tried to determine the factors conditioning this differing perception. To what extent does the complaint depend on the disturbing environmental factor and to what extent on the characteristics of the individual? Studies have been carried out to relate sex, age, occupation, social group, education, and attitudes to the perception of the trouble source (25). Such studies are more than theoretical exercises since they contribute to the legal and regulatory basis for the control of sanitary nuisances.

Some findings of these studies have indicated that:

a. People who are generally content in their residential area (i.e., adequately adapted) are less likely to complain about a specific environmental defect than people who are not satisfied with their residential area. In studying reaction to airplane noise, Norwegian investigators found that people who have a positive attitude to aircraft (i.e., users who are familiar with flying) had a tendency to be less troubled by airplane noise than the others. A caution is always necessary, since this finding has not been reproducible in other countries.

b. Women complain more than men about environmental hazards such as dust, smog, odor, etc. This is quite understandable, since they commonly are subject to a more intensive and prolonged exposure at home, while men are off to their occupations. It has been theorized that women are more physiologically sensitive to noise and other environmental hazards. For instance, hearing in women becomes less impaired with age than in men. This point, however, requires further investigation, and needs to be related to other evidence of women's state of adaptation.

c. Though the theoretical evidence is sparse, practical experiences support a hypothesis that complaints and environmental annoyance may be conditioned by the special relationships between the individuals exposed to and the individuals causing the nuisance. There is the familiar case of increased sensitivity to the nuisance when there is a problem between neighbors. At the other extreme, there is the evidence that people who derive their living from a plant causing air pollution are less troubled than others by the air pollution nuisance emanating from this plant.

Sociologists are particularly interested in the possibility that the social setting is related to a special individual sensibility or individual adaptability to external environmental factors. The hypothesis has been advanced that the person living in a particularly oppressive social setting is more sensitive generally to the stress of the totality of external environmental factors.

If attitude is an important background variable in the genesis of complaints, then several approaches are possible:

a. the specific deleterious environmental factor can be modified. This is the current approach;

b. the attitude of the person toward those responsible for the nuisance can be altered (the public relations campaigns of a number of companies illustrate this approach). The shortcoming of this solution is apparent; and,

c. the totality of environmental and social conditions influencing general well-being in the neighboorhood can be improved.

This latter approach supposes that there is synergistic action between external environmental conditions; i.e., one environmental stress adds to the intensity of another in such a way that the combined effect is greater than the sum of stresses. This point, of course, has implications for the need to ameliorate the total urban condition rather than solutions in tight disciplinary compartments. Environmental health specialists may learn from sociologists, psychologists, and the mental health profession about the interface between mind, attitude, and preferences on one hand, and the physical environment, on the other hand. Pervasive urban annoyances are particularly important and deserve a new look. The investigation of the genesis and distribution of such urban annoyances has significance for the interrelationship between social organization and environmental health, and for adequate individual adaptation.

Epidemiologic Contributions

Although there is no intention to convey the impression that control of the physical environment is all that is needed to provide good adaptation for people, it is worthwhile spelling out some of the ways in which the adequate adaptation of many people might be protected or improved, and the occurrence of adaptational inadequacies prevented to some extent through environmental control. Recent epidemiological studies such as the one in midtown Manhattan (26), in rural Stirling County (15), in a small town in Sweden (27), and in the State of Texas (28), produce convincing evidence that the bio-socio-cultural environment determines, to a surprisingly large extent, who it is that develops psychiatric disorder.

In metropolitan New York, the principal factor appeared to be socio-economic status, which quite obviously affects the biological necessities and determines the possibility of securing adequate amounts of the psychological and social needs listed. In rural Stirling County, socioeconomic status was also important, but even more important was the degree of sociocultural integration of the small communities in which the subjects lived. In well-integrated communities, even poor people had quite good mental health; whereas in the disintegrated communities, which share many features (other than size) with city slums, even the few prosperous residents had poor mental health. In Texas, Jaco found strong influences by ethnic affiliation and by length of residence in the State upon the prevalence rate and the type of psychotic illness.

If, indeed, social environment makes so much difference, what evidence is there that improvement in the social environment actually affects mental health? Unfortunately, most efforts to bring about social improvements have not been accompanied by adequate (if any) mental health research, and conversely, little mental health research has been accompanied by action programs. There are, however, two bits of evidence which hint, at least, that changes in the environment, whether spontaneous or contrived, may favorably influence mental health. These findings will be briefly described.

One of these events (29) took place in Stirling County in a small slum-like community which was first surveyed in 1952 and was found to show a high prevalence of maladaptive symptoms, as well as general poverty, scanty education, high intra-group hostility, little evidence of affectionate feelings between people, and a general state of anomie. The only intentional effort to influence the social environment was brought to bear by an adult educator and by a teacher who succeeded him. The educator's first step was to try to get people out of their homes and into some kind of group setting so that they could begin to interact with one another and be led, perhaps, into some constructive group endeavor. He began by showing them movies in the local one-room school, then encouraging them to choose the next week's movie, finally requesting that they contribute half the sum required to wire the school for electricity. The teacher took over by getting the women to hold community bingo parties to finance new school desks, and eventually taught them how to utilize their votes to enlist the aid of the larger society in their behalf, in this case so that they could get their children accepted into the consolidated school district in the interest of better education.

In addition, an economic arrangement was established, without any outside suggestion, in which individuals or couples would go to a distant industrial center for six months or a year, work in a factory, save their money, and return home to invest it in home improvements. Homes began to take on an altogether different appearance as they were repaired or enlarged and even landscaped to some extent. Another economic boost, in which a job offer was accompanied by the opportunity to purchase electrical equipment on credit, brought this disadvantaged group very nearly into even step with the surrounding, non-disadvantaged population. When the community's mental health was resurveyed in 1962, it had improved to such an extent that it was approximately the same as the whole county. All the sociocultural indicators had also improved in the direction of the county average, and there was good evidence that social interaction was frequent and friendly within the community. Not enough is known at this time to say which of the various things that happened was the most important. It seems probable that no one event was crucial, but rather that it was the complex—which included economic betterment, the emergence of social supports, and a greatly improved self-image, due in part to a demonstrated abiltiy to compete in the industrial world—that made the difference.

The other situation became apparent when an attempt was made to compare the prevalence of psychiatric disorder and various sociocultural features of a small town in Sweden with a small town in Stirling County (27). The Stirling County town showed the same inverse relationship of mental health to socioeconomic status as did the whole county. Dohrenwend (30) states that 14 of 18 studies, in which measures of psychiatric disorder are related to socioeconomic status, show the same relationship. The Swedish town, however, showed a reverse relationship in which the highest prevalence of psychiatric disorder accompanied highest economic status, and lowest prevalence was found amoung the lowest economic group. The explanation that has been advanced for this finding is that Swedish social reforms of the 20th Century have done much to counteract the disadvantages, insecurities, and opprobrium commonly associated with lowest status in Western civilizations.

These two examples suggest strongly that improvement in the *social* environment probably does have a favorable effect on mental health (adaptive status). What extensions of these findings can be made to a wider range of environmental influences? Still thinking of the social environment, it seems quite clear that the heavy migration to cities, without regard to social arrangements which might preserve social supports, must upset the psychological and social equilibrium quite drastically. Country people, accustomed to knowing and interacting with their neighbors on a familiar basis, find themselves in a mass of unknown persons who have also left behind their social supports. Fear and caution lead to withdrawn behavior, with no one wanting to make a first move, and each family group surrounding itself with something of a wall. There is not the same opportunity for escape from people into fields and woods in the city as in the country. The chief escape available is to disregard the people in the immediate environment, or to indulge in alcohol or drugs. Soon a feeling develops that whatever happens is the fault of some of these strangers, plus a conviction that there is no one who will help in a crisis. While definitive studies which supply all the links of the casual chain are still in the future, findings with regard to elevated blood pressure suggest that the notions expressed here are more than a fantasy.

On the physical side, overcrowding because of high rents, poor ventilation, and inadequate heating, supplemented by deficient diets, due to low income plus ignorance of nutritional needs, no arrangements for people to get together socially, and no money for anything but bare survival, puts people in a state of uneasiness and tension which predisposes them to a myriad of diseases (31, 32). If the wage earners fall ill, everything is that much worse.

Wilner (33), in his study of 1,000 families in Baltimore, found that there was better social psychological adjustment of families who were housed in low-rent housing projects than among similar families residing in substandard dwelling units. In general, the families living in the low-rent housing projects showed less social disorganization and more neighborly interaction of a mutually supportive kind.

Effects of Environmental Defects

The esthetic effect of squalor upon the human personality has never been measured precisely. Such deprivation may be endured if it is not a permanent condition, but when it lasts for generations there is almost bound to be a demoralization. When there is added the outpourings of irritant gases, the diminution in sunshine, the high and unending level of noise, the high count of particulate matter in the air, which settles indoors and out-of-doors into a crunchy layer, the impossibility to entertain friends in the overcrowded apartment, or to find any place where one can visit informally and pleasantly, one wonders why anyone stays in the city. The reason, of course, is the comparative availability of work which is needed to provide the money for fundamental necessities as well as for the many desirable items seen on television or in store windows, or on the person of the neighbor. Country living may provide more space and beauty, more sunshine and cleaner air, but it is not sufficient for modern wants.

Environmental scientists and city planners could probably accomplish considerable reforms that would favorably affect the mental health of city dwellers if they would think in terms of satisfying as many as possible of the basic psychosocial needs which we have listed. The reason for cities is circular—people crowd in because there are factory jobs there, and more factories come because there are many workers available. From the viewpoint of human needs, it would be better (as many people have suggested) to disperse factories and to let them attract smaller numbers of people, who will be less damaged by less intense urbanization, because it will be somewhat easier for them to reestablish the necessary social matrix. The effect of such a change on air and water pollution could be merely to disseminate the contaminants over a larger area. On the other hand, adequately enforced current techniques could be expected to control the situation to a larger extent than is possible in the urban setting.

Two of the more pressing problems in the United States today are poverty and family disorganization. Both problems have dimensions that have special import to the environmentalist and the mental health specialist. Some researchers have claimed that there must be a causal relationship between substandard housing and family and social disorganization in view of the high incidence of both in slum areas. However, as long ago as 1936, James Ford (34) concluded that both were simply parts of the "syndrome of poverty." Available data are insufficient to prove either point, but the syndrome of poverty has gained general currency. Of principal importance is not how these facts are related, but that some form of relationship, direct or indirect, exists.

Schorr (35) points out that there are three types of evidence of the effects of the residential environment on attitudes and behavior. The most prevalent is the personal or case observation in which knowledge is gained at firsthand. The second is statistically correlated data on the relationship between an element of the environment and human behavior. The third is comparison of behavior and attitudes of people in different environmental circumstances. Schorr concludes that "though the evidence is scattered, taken as a whole, it is substantial. The type of housing occupied influences health, behavior and attitude, particularly if the housing is desperately inadequate." Gunnar Myrdal (36) wrote, " any common sense evaluation will tell us that the causation, in part, goes from poor housing to bad moral, mental, and physical health." Cannan (37) is credited with concluding that "filthy environments may make us mentally ill before they make us physically sick."

The National Advisory Commission on Civil Disorders (38) expressed itself on the inadequacy of the housing environment of the Negro population in the United States. It called upon all the American people to put a stop to the social and economic decay of our major cities. Some analysts believe that the substandard physical environment of the Negro ghetto, coupled with general social unrest, created sufficient frustrations and irritations to be blamed as a partial cause of some of the civil disorders.

ENVIRONMENTAL HEALTH SPECIALISTS' RESPONSIBILITY

The challenges that face environmental health specialists today in an urbanized society can be grouped into four broad categories according to the Task Force on Environmental Health and Related Problems (10). They are:
1. controlling pollution at its source;
2. reducing hazards;
3. converting wastes to use; and
4. improving the esthetic value of man's surroundings.

To develop solutions to the many individual problems that are grouped in the above classification requires a more adequate understanding of ordinary human behavior than has been exhibited by environmental health specialists in the past. The many lost battles of environmental control during the past few decades, such as the difficulty of developing and enforcing desirable minimum standards of water quality in rivers, streams and lakes, and the impossibility in some communities of instituting fluoridation programs, are measurements of the inadequacy shown by present environmentalists to understand social forces. At the most fundamental level the environmental health specialist must understand the importance of culture socialization in determining how people perceive what goes on in the environment and its "good" and "bad" import. He must comprehend that what seems to him a purely technical problem may have social and emotional implications to the public of a far-reaching nature, and that his success in dealing with the technical aspects will be strongly influenced by his ability to discover these implications in advance. He must, moreover, learn about social process, about governmental mechanisms and about how his own type of activity affects, and is affected by these considerations.

It has been said that environmental health is more closely related to overall physical and social planning than any of the other health fields. The environmental health professions are concerned about population density and the impact that density may have on the provision of acceptable air and water, pollution control, and the maintenance of a satisfactory environment. In dealing with such impacts, the social environment itself is a variable that must be measured, evaluated, and modified.

As we have said, environmental health workers have been largely component-oriented in their approach to problem-solving. Therefore, in dealing with environmental pollution control, the interrelation of the social environment with the biological, chemical, and physical environments has not been sufficiently taken into account. It should be noted, however, that there is a growing roster of social scientists concerned with the physical environment. Some experts suggest that a possible reason for the increasing levels of effort required for control is the inadequacy of the component-oriented approach to provide a solution. These experts suggest that system-oriented approaches will provide more effective solutions. The system-oriented approach to environmental pollution control must include the social system if the analysis and solution are to be comprehensive.

Concomitant with almost all modifications of the physical environment are changes in the social environment, some of which are for the betterment, others for the worsening of the human situation. Therefore, the environmentalist should become acquainted with human ecology and should learn to understand the interactions of the biological, chemical, physical, and social environments with each other.

The environmentalist is already deeply involved in social engineering, though he usually does not see his activity in this light. A modicum of this is essential in his bringing about almost any successful environmental change for the better health of a group of people. Since this has not been seen, typically, as any of his business, he neither understands nor accepts the implications of the results of his activity on the social and cultural aspects of the life of the group he is presumably helping. As for the notion that his activity bears even the remotest relationship to human adaptation or mental health, he would probably shudder at the very thought. Since most environmentalists, however, are themselves part of some human group (or several), it should not be too difficult to open their eyes a bit regarding the matters just discussed.

CURRICULUM FOR ENVIRONMENTAL SPECIALISTS

Desirable inputs to the educational program for environmental specialists include:

a. knowledge of how to stimulate political action, influence public decisionmaking, mold public opinion;
b. how to determine attitudes;
c. how to recognize the social and psychological patterns of the public being served;
d. a view of environmental science as a means to an end, not an end in itself, in which the taking account of public attitudes and desires will facilitate the tasks of the environmentalists;
e. an orientation regarding social and cultural organization in general;
f. the socio-cultural-political-economic implications of public health and environmental protection activities;

g. the effect of particular environmental programs or endeavors on the people being served;

h. an understanding of the available resources of mental health which are applicable to practitioners in the fields of environmental sciences and engineering.

For courses dealing primarily with environmental health, it is probably better to have the mental health input teaching done by environmental sciences and engineering faculty who have acquainted themselves with the required materials. Alternatives are to have consultation by a mental health expert, to have a joint environmental health/mental health teaching team, or to have a mental health faculty member responsible for presenting the mental health content. The best plan would seem to be to have a mental health consultant help with the planning, and an environmental health faculty member do the teaching.

The long-range objective is to have the entire environmental health faculty appreciate and actively support the notion of the importance of human factors in environmental health. One way to do this might be to persuade the faculty to take part in discussions of human ecology, which is recognized as a concern of environmental scientists. Points raised in such discussions by the environmentalists could then be taken up and elaborated and related to the social environment.

Human behavior content for environmental specialists could be provided by means of the following types of experiences:

a. an assignment for students to spend some time in a blighted central area of a city, studying the social and environmental problems and interviewing a number of residents of the area on matters such as housing conditions, garbage and refuse disposal, recreation, traffic, noise, etc.;

b. instruction in the social aspects of city planning;

c. study of the Hawthorne experiment (39) and other more recent industrial-environmental social-psychological studies;

d. studies of case histories of efforts to introduce environmental sanitation programs into various cultural groups (40);

e. a stimulated project in health-focused social change with an environmentalist in association with a public health administrator, a public health nurse, and a social scientist;

f. attendance at meetings of town, city, or county officials when environmenal matters, including housing and recreation, are discussed;

g. participation in local health department environmental health projects in which most of the public health specialists in the department participate, providing expert advice and assistance as appropriate; and,

h. instruction in consultation technique, followed by supervised consultation assignments.

All of the preceding activities should be preceded by lectures and readings, and followed by discussions.

SUMMARY

In the past, the practice of environmental health has been concerned largely with only the biological, chemical, and physical components of human life, omitting the social components. However, a comprehensive approach to environmental health must include the social environment of man and his adjustments to it. Mental health, as defined, is a state of adequate adaption to the biological-chemical-physical and social-psychological environment in which man resides.

Good adaptation (or good mental health) is dependent therefore upon many factors. Improvement or protection of adaptation can be facilitated to some degree through environmental control. Many of the current health problems, such as environmental pollution, crowding and congestion, noise, odor, etc., pose serious threats not only to physical health but also to mental health and social well-being. While the evidence to support the hypothesis that changing the physical environment of man affects his mental health is fragmentary, collectively these data suggest that improvement in the environment, either spontaneous or contrived, has a favorable influence on the adaptive status of people.

Two of the pressing problems of the United States today are poverty and family disorganization, both of which involve environmental control and adaptation. Solutions to these problems must involve an integration of the concepts and principles of environmental health and mental health and should be developed through joint physical and social planning.

REFERENCES

1. *Urban Sprawl and Health.* Report of the 1958 Health Forum, National Health Council, New York, 1959.
2. *Proceedings : Conference on "Man Versus Environment."* Edited by H. A. Faber and M. H. Peak, California Institute of Technology, Pasadena, Calif., 1959.
3. *Report on Environmental Health Problems.* Hearings before the Subcommittee of the Committee on Appropriations, House of Representatives, 86th Congr., 2d sess., Washington, D.C., 1960.
4. *Report of the Committee on Environmental Health Problems to the Surgeon General.* U.S. Department of Health, Education, and Welfare, Public Health Service, Washington, D.C., 1962.
5. *Restoring the Quality of Our Environment.* Report of the Environmental Pollution Panel, President's Science Advisory Committee, The White House, Washington, D. C., 1963.
6. *Environmental Determinants of Community Well-Being.* Pan American

Health Organization, Washington, D.C., 1965.

7. *The Adequacy of Technology for Pollution Abatement, Volume I.* Hearings before the Subcommittee on Science, Research, and Development of the Committee on Science and Astronautics, House of Representatives, 89th Congr., 2d sess., Washington, D.C. 1966.

8. *The Adequacy of Technology for Pollution Abatement., Volume II.* Hearings before the Subcommittee on Science, Research, and Development of the Committee on Science and Astronautics, House of Representatives, 89th Cong., 2d sess., Washington, D.C., 1966.

9. *Waste Management and Control.* National Academy of Sciences—National Research Council, Publication 1400, Washington, D.C., 1966.

10. *A Strategy for a Livable Environment.* A Report to the Secretary of Health, Education, and Welfare by the Task Force on Environmental Health and Related Problems, Washington, D.C., 1967.

11. In testimony presented to the Subcommittee of the Committee on Appropriations, House of Representatives, U.S. Congress, March 8, 1960, at a special hearing on the problems of environmental health.

12. *Changing Environmental Hazards. Challenges to Community Health.* Report of the Task Force on Environmental Health, National Commission on Community Health Services, Public Affairs Press, Washington, D.C., 1967.

13. Bosch, H.M. The teaching of environmental health. *Public Health Reports,* 76 : 155–158, 1961.

14. Leighton, A.H. *My Name is Legion.* New York : Basic Books, 1959.

15. Leighton, D.C., et al. *The Character of Danger.* New York : Basic Books, 1963.

16. Cassel, J.C., and Tyroler, H.A. Epidemiological studies of culture change: I. Health status and recency of industrialization. *Archives of Environmental Health,* 3 : 25–33, July 1961.

16a. Health consequences of culture change: II. The effect of urbanization on coronary health mortality in rural residents. *J. Chronic Dis.,* 17 : 167–177, February 1964.

17. Leighton, D.C., and Cline, N.F. The public health nurse as a mental health resource. *In:* Weaver, T., ed., *Essays on Medical Anthropology.* Athens, Ga.: University of Georgia Press, 1968.

18. Jarrett, H. ed. *Environmental Quality in a Growing Economy,* published for Resources for the Future, Inc., by The Johns Hopkins Press, Baltimore, 1966.

19. Fisher, J. L. The natural environment. *Annals of the American Academy of Political and Social Science,* 371 : 127–140, 1967.

20. U.S. Outdoor Recreation Resources Review Commission. *Outdoor Recreation for America,* Washington, U.S. Government Printing Office, 1962.

21. U.S. Department of Health, Education, and Welfare. *Community Perception of Air Quality.* Public Health Service Publication No. 999–AP–10. Cincinnati, 1965.

22. U.S. Department of Health, Education, and Welfare. *Public Awareness and Concern with Air Pollution in the St. Louis Metropolitan Area.* Washington Public Health Service, Division of Air Pollution, 1965.

23. Van Arsdol, M. D.; Sabagh, G.; and Francesca, A. Reality and the Perception of Environmental Hazards. *J. of Health and Human Behavior,* 5 : 144–153, 1964.

24. Kates, R. W., and Wohlwill, J. F., eds. Man's response to the physical environment. *Journal of Social Issues,* 22 : 1–141, 1966.
25. Jonsson, E. Annoyance reactions to external environmental factors in different sociological groups. *Acta Sociologia,* 7 : 229–261, 1964.
26. Srole, L. et al. *Mental health in the Metropolis,* New York : McGraw Hill, 1962.
27. Leighton, D. C., et al. Psychiatric disorder in a Swedish and a Canadian community. (Mimeo in preparation.)
28. Jaco, E. G. *The Social Epidemiology of Mental Disorder.* New York: Russell Sage Foundation, 1960.
29. Leighton, A. H. Poverty and social change. *Scientific American.* 212 : 21–27, May 1965.
30. Dohrenwend, B. D. The problem of validity in field studies of psychological disorder. *Journal Abnor. Psychol.,* 70 : 52–69, 1965.
31. Hall, E. T. Proxemics: The study of man's spatial relations. In *Man's Image in Medicine and Anthropology.* New York, 1963.
32. Reisman, D. *The Lonely Crowd.* New Haven: Yale Press, 1950.
33. Wilner, D. M., et al. *The Housing Environment and Family Life,* Baltimore: The Johns Hopkins Press, 1962.
34. Ford, J. *Slums and Housing.* Cambridge: Harvard University Press, 1936.
35. Schorr, A. L. *Slums and Social Insecurity.* Research Report No. 1, Social Security Administration, Department of Health, Education, and Welfare, U.S. Government Printing Office, Washington, 1963.
36. Myrdal, G. *An American Dilemma.* New York: Harper and Brothers, 1944, vol. 1.
37. Cannan, R. K. The experimental City. *Daedalus,* 96 : 1132, 1967.
38. *Report of the National Advisory Commission on Civil Disorders,* New York: Bantam Books, 1968.
39. Roethlisberger, F. A. *Management and Morale.* Cambridge: Harvard University Press, 1944.
40. Paul, B. *Health, Culture and Community.* New York: Russell Sage Foundation, 1965.

BIBLIOGRAPHY

Arensberg, C.M., and Niehoff, A.H. *Introducing Social Change.* Chicago : Aldine, 1964.
Back, K.W. *Slums, Projects and People: Social-Psychological Problems of Relocation in Puerto Rico.* Durham : Duke University Press, 1962.
Chapin, F. S. Some housing factors related to mental hygiene. *American Journal of Public Health,* 41 : 839-842, July 1951.
Calhoun, J.B. Population density and social pathology. *Scientific American,* February 1962.
Dubos, R. *Man Adapting.* New Haven : Yale University Press, 1965.
Francis, T., Jr. Biological aspects of environment. *Industrial Medicine and Surgery,* 30 : 374, September 1961.
Fried, M. Some sources of residential satisfaction in an urban slum. *Journal of American Institute of Planners,* 27 : 305-315, November 1961.
Gans, H.J. The human implications of current redevelopment and relocation

planning. *Journal of American Institute of Planners,* 25 : 15-25, February 1959.

Goffman, E. *The Presentation of the Self in Everyday Life.* New York, 1959.

Hall, E.T. *The Hidden Dimension.* New York : Doubleday, 1966.

Hartman, C.W. Social values and housing orientation. *The Journal of Social Issues,* 19 (2) : 118-130, April 1963.

Lemkau, P.V. *Mental Hygiene in Public Health.* 2d. ed. New York : McGraw Hill Company, 1955.

Lynch, K. The city as environment. *Scientific American,* 213 : 209, 1965.

Malpass, L. F., ed. *Social Behavior.* New York : McGraw-Hill, 1965. (A programed instruction book.)

McDermott, W. Air pollution and public health. *Scientific American,* October 1961.

Ratcliffe, H.L. Editorial—environmental factors and coronary diseases. *Circulation,* 27 : 481-482, April 1963.

Ratcliffe, H.L., and Snyder, R.L. Patterns of disease, controlled population and experimental design. *Circulation,* 26 : 1352-1357, December 1962.

Roscow, I. The social effects of the physical environment. *Journal American Institute of Planners,* 27 : 127-133, 1961.

Wolman, A. The metabolism of cities. *Scientific American,* 213 : 179, September, 1965.

Woodbury, C., ed. *Urban Redevelopment: Problems and Practices.* Chicago: University of Chicago Press, 1953.

II. UNDERSTANDING

AIR POLLUTION

Air

INTRODUCTION

The air which envelopes the Earth is the life-supporting medium in which man lives, just as water is the medium in which fish exist. It is required in the combustion of fuel whereby man generates heat and power. It is used in manufacturing processes and service activities, such as chemical and biological oxidation processes, air cooling, and spray painting. The air supply is limited and must be reused. In the course of natural and artificial ventilation, used air, along with any waste products, mixes with the surrounding ambient air which is thereby polluted. Many waste products in the air are damaging, both to man and various elements of his environment. Fortunately, polluted air is subject to natural cleansing and rejuvenating. When these systems become overloaded and the tolerance of man and his environment is exceeded, man must either suffer the consequences or initiate action to preclude resulting damage and loss.

Air pollution control has been carried out from time to time and to various levels of sophistication for hundreds of years. But, until the relatively recent episodes of death-dealing smog in London, the Meuse Valley of Belgium, and Donora, Pennsylvania, such actions were generally for the purpose of lessening a nuisance. Today there is a substantial and growing realization that the ecology is changing rapidly and that man's existence as a species of this planet is threatened. Damaging air pollution is the principal result and indicator of this change. Air pollution is a regional problem. County-wide and multi-county programs have been established in various parts of the United States in recognition of this fact. Mounting effective air quality management is complex, difficult, and expensive. It involves major considerations and actions in the technologic, sociologic, economic, political, and legal arenas. Nevertheless, society has deemed that air pollution control must be achieved in order to promote man's total health and well-being.

The mission of air pollution control agencies is to reduce to a minimum the

Excerpts from: *Environmental Health Planning,* U.S. Department of Health, Education and Welfare. Public Health Service Publication 2120, Bureau of Community Environmental Management, 1971.

amount of pollutants emitted from existing sources and to minimize the introduction of additional pollutants from new sources. Control programs should be operated as efficiently and effectively as possible. Under the complex and difficult circumstances that prevail, a thoughtful and effective planning effort is demanded.

PROBLEMS

Despite the spectacular increased effort in the 1960's to control air pollution, the best that can be said, in most areas of the Nation, is that they've barely been able to hold the line. Both population and standard of living continue to increase and with these there is a resulting increase in the production and use of goods and services. Each year there are more automobiles, more power-generating facilities, more new chemical compounds, more manufacturing plants, more use of fertilizers and pesticides—all resulting in more sources of atmospheric emissions. Air pollution is considered to be a major factor in respiratory ailments such as lung cancer, emphysema, chronic bronchitis, and common colds. It appears to be a factor in heart disease and abnormal human behavior. It causes eye irritation. Air pollution causes economic loss due to damage to vegetation, animals, materials and visibility. It reduces agricultural productivity and reduces the salability of fruits, flowers and vegetables. It adversely affects normal growth and function of domestic animals. It damages paint and erodes metals, masonry, and air sculptures. It fades and deteriorates fabrics, and damages the connections and switches of electrical systems. It reduces visibility and thus spoils or obliterates vistas, causes airplane and vehicular accidents, delays airplane schedules, and reduces real property values.

Air pollutants are in the form of solid and liquid particulates and gases. They occur in the air in varying particle sizes, concentrations, and combinations, and problems result after anywhere from short to long exposure times, depending upon the nature of the pollutant and the sensitivity of the receptor. Odor problems occur almost instantaneously when a very low concentration of a single gaseous pollutant comes in contact with the human nose, while noticeable damage to a stone sculpture may require years of exposure to relatively high concentrations of sulfur dioxide, particulates, and humidity. Significant problems for a small area may be limited to those caused by emissions from a single "point" source, such as a smelter, power plant, paper mill or chemical manufacturing plant. For regional areas with an urban core, however, air pollution is caused by the emissions from a large number of sources, both stationary and mobile. Identification and quantification of the problem requires an evaluation of the pollutant source-receptor system of the area, considering such factors as the nature and location of pollutant sources, quantities of source emissions, topography, meteorology, and measured and predicted levels of air quality. Such evaluations serve as the basis for subsequent monitoring, emission inventory, and regulatory activities.

Assessment of the causes and effects requires a wide range of capability of technical personnel, gas and particulate monitoring equipment, and techniques and equipment for measuring damage. Control agency equipment for gases, for example, ranges anywhere from simple qualitative samplers wherein the change in color of a chemically treated piece of paper identifies the presence of a relatively high concentration of a gaseous pollutant, to a sophisticated volumetric gas chromatograph which "reads out" the identity and very low concentration of a gas in an air sample brought to the laboratory. The level of sophistication needed depends upon the degree and nature of the problem and the amount and type of regulatory authority the agency possesses.

Air Pollution

We tend to view air pollution as a recently discovered phenomenon. But since the dawn of the industrial revolution, people in many communities have endured levels of smoke pollution that would be held intolerable today. In the last half of the 19th century, a surprising number of aroused citizen groups protested the smoke-laden air of London. But their protests were lost in the overwhelming clamor for industrial development at any price.

Progress in the United States was no more heartening. Chicago and Cincinnati passed smoke control laws in 1881. By 1912, 23 of the 28 American cities with populations over 200,000 had passed similar laws. But still there was little dent made in air pollution.

In the 1930's, 1940's, and 1950's smoke pollution reached its zenith in the United States, especially in Eastern and Midwestern industrial cities. The public outcry against these conditions resulted in the enactment of improved smoke pollution legislation, its partial enforcement, and a visible improvement in the air of some industrial cities. These local control efforts focused primarily on cutting down smoke from fossil fuels, particularly coal. The fortunate advent of diesel engines in place of steam locomotives and the increased use of gas as a fuel for space heating also helped cut back air pollution in that era.

The Donora disaster in Pennsylvania in 1948 pricked the conscience of the Nation, but the experience of Los Angeles beginning in that same decade was a more certain sign of the complex air pollution problem which now confronts cities throughout the world. When the citizens of Los Angeles began to complain of smog, few people suspected that air pollution was a great deal more than just smoke. Los Angeles used virtually none of the fuels primarily responsible for the smoke problems of cities elsewhere; yet smog appeared and worsened. Dr. Arie J. Haagen-Smit, of the California Institute of Technology, finally pinpointed the principal sources of photochemical smog in Los Angeles—hydrocarbons and nitrogen oxides from automobile exhausts. Smog was at first thought to be a phenomenon amplified by local weather conditions and limited to Los Angeles.

Excerpts from *Environmental Quality*, The First Annual Report of the Council on Environmental Quality, August, 1970.

Today, however, most major cities are afflicted to some degree by photo-chemical smog as well as by other forms of air pollution.

Air pollution is for the most part a phenomenon of urban living that occurs when the capacity of the air to dilute the pollutants is overburdened. Population and industrial growth and a high degree of dependence on the motor vehicle cause new gaseous and particulate emissions to complement, interact with, and further complicate the traditional ones.

When the first Federal air pollution control legislation was passed in 1955, there were no viable ongoing State programs at all. There was little interest in the scientific community, and the public, by and large, equated air pollution with coal smoke and considered smog a problem unique to Los Angeles. It is no wonder that air pollution is regarded as a recently discovered phenomenon.

POLLUTANTS AND THEIR SOURCES

Five main classes of pollutants are pumped into the air over the United States, totaling more than 200 million tons per year. These are summarized in table 1 for 1968, the latest year for which data are available for making estimates.

Transportation—particularly the automobile—is the greatest source of air pollution. It accounts for 42 percent of all pollutants by weight. It produces major portions not only of carbon monoxide but of hydrocarbons and nitrogen oxides.

Table 1.—Estimated Nationwide Emissions, 1968

[In millions of tons per year]

Source	Carbon mon-oxide	Partic-ulates	Sulfur oxides	Hydro-carbons	Nitrogen oxides	Total
Transportation-------------------	63.8	1.2	0.8	16.6	8.1	90.5
Fuel combustion in stationary sources--	1.9	8.9	24.4	.7	10.0	45.9
Industrial processes---------------	9.7	7.5	7.3	4.6	.2	29.3
Solid waste disposal---------------	7.8	1.1	.1	1.6	.6	11.2
Miscellaneous[1]-------------------	16.9	9.6	.6	8.5	1.7	37.3
Total	100.1	28.3	33.2	32.0	20.6	214.2

[1]Primarily forest fires, agricultural burning, coal waste fires.
Source: NAPCA Inventory of Air Pollutant Emissions, 1970.

Carbon monoxide (CO) is a colorless, odorless, poisonous gas, slightly lighter than air, that is produced by the incomplete burning of the carbon in fuels. Carbon monoxide emissions can be prevented by supplying enough air to insure complete combustion. When this occurs, carbon dioxide, a natural constituent of the atmosphere, is produced instead of carbon monoxide.

Almost two-thirds of the carbon monoxide emitted comes from internal combustion engines, and the overwhelming bulk of that comes from gasoline-powered motor vehicles.

Particulate matter includes particles of solid or liquid substances in a very wide range of sizes, from those that are visible as soot and smoke to particles too small to detect except under an electron microscope. Particulates may be so small that they remain in the air for long periods and can be transported great distances by the winds. They are produced primarily by stationary fuel combustion (31 percent) and industrial processes (27 percent). Forest fires and other miscellaneous sources account for 34 percent.

There are established techniques for controlling particulates from a boiler stack or from a waste air stream—among them filtering, washing, centrifugal separation, and electrostatic precipitation. These work well for most of the particles, but complete removal, especially of the very finest particles, is technically and economically difficult.

Sulfur oxides (SOx) are acrid, corrosive, poisonous gases produced when fuel containing sulfur is burned. Electric utilities and industrial plants are its principal producers since their most abundant fuels are coal and oil, which contain sulfur as an impurity. The burning of coal produces about 60 percent of all sulfur oxides emissions, oil about 14 percent, and industrial processes that use sulfur 22 percent. Most of the coal is burned in electric power generation plants. About two-thirds of the Nation's sulfur oxides are emitted in urban areas, where industry and population are concentrated. And seven industrial States in the Northeast account for almost half of the national total of sulfur oxides. In rural areas, however, sulfur oxides sources may be large industrial plants, smelters, or power plants. Any one of these may throw out several hundred thousand tons of sulfur oxides in a year.

Government agencies and industry have sought to reduce sulfur oxide emissions in three ways: switching to low sulfur fuels (those with less than 1 percent sulfur), removing sulfur from fuels entirely, and removing sulfur oxides from the combustion gases.

Hydrocarbons (HC), like carbon monoxide, represent unburned and wasted fuel. Unlike carbon monoxide, gaseous hydrocarbons at concentrations normally found in the atmosphere are not toxic, but they are a major pollutant because of their role in forming photochemical smog. More than half the estimated 32 million tons of hydrocarbons produced each year comes from transportation sources, mainly gasoline-fueled vehicles. Another 27 percent comes from miscellaneous burning and 14 percent from industrial processes. About 60 percent is produced in urban areas, largely because there are more automobiles.

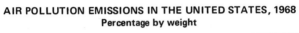

AIR POLLUTION EMISSIONS IN THE UNITED STATES, 1968
Percentage by weight

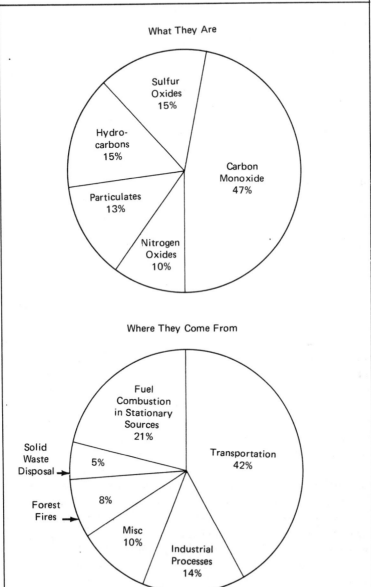

What They Are

Sulfur Oxides 15%

Hydro-carbons 15%

Particulates 13%

Nitrogen Oxides 10%

Carbon Monoxide 47%

Where They Come From

Fuel Combustion in Stationary Sources 21%

Solid Waste Disposal → 5%

Forest Fires → 8%

Misc 10%

Transportation 42%

Industrial Processes 14%

Source: National Air Pollution Control Administration, HEW.

Nitrogen oxides (NOx) are produced when fuel is burned at very high temperatures. Stationary combustion plants produce 49 percent of the nitrogen oxide emissions; transportation vehicles, 39 percent; and all other sources, 12 percent.

Internal combustion engines operate at very high temperatures, and so do efficient, large electric power and industrial boilers. Nitrogen that is ordinarily inert combines with oxygen in high temperature flames and tends to stay combined if the exhaust gases are cooled too quickly. The control of NOx from stationary sources requires careful adjustment of flame and stack gas temperatures. Control of nitrogen oxides from automobiles is more difficult because reducing other pollutants can increase the output of NOx.

Under the influence of sunlight, nitrogen oxides combine with gaseous hydrocarbons to form a complex variety of secondary pollutants called *photochemical oxidants.* These oxidants, together with solid and liquid particles in the air, make up what is commonly known as smog. The photochemical oxidant family of pollutants includes, among others, ozone, an unstable, toxic form of oxygen; nitrogen dioxide; peroxyacyl nitrates; aldehydes; and acrolein. In air they can cause eye and lung irritation, damage to vegetation, offensive odor, and thick haze.

WHAT AIR POLLUTION DOES

Air pollution adversely affects man and his environment in many ways. It soils his home and interferes with the growth of plants and shrubs. It diminishes the value of his agricultural products. It obscures his view and adds unpleasant smells to his environment. Most important, it endangers his health.

The extent of air pollution depends heavily on how weather disposes of the pollutants. The ability of the atmosphere to dilute and disperse them is limited to two factors—wind speed and the depth in the atmosphere to which air near the surface can be mixed. Although considerable variation occurs from day to day in the extent to which these factors disperse air pollution, the same patterns tend to repeat themselves over months or years. On some few days in a year, strong winds and highly unstable atmospheric conditions may disperse even the heaviest blanket of pollution. On many other days, weak winds and highly stable conditions let small quantities of pollutants accumulate and build up to serious proportions. Between these extremes, variations in weather conditions create varying levels of pollution over a given area.

Many cities lie in natural basins at the confluence of rivers, around bays, or in flat areas backed against mountains. Such basins are natural gathering places for low-lying masses of warm air, which trap pollutants in the familiar phenomenon known as an "inversion." However, even communities more favorably located increasingly find that atmospheric conditions limit the amount of air available as a dumping place for pollutants.

... to Human Health

The most important effect of air pollution is its threat to human health. Acute episodes of pollution in London, New York, and other cities have been marked by dramatic increases in death and illness rates, especially among the elderly and those with preexisting respiratory or cardiac conditions.

The incident most familiar to Americans occurred in 1948 in Donora, an industrial town in the mountains of western Pennsylvania. Almost half of the town's 14,000 inhabitants fell ill; 20 died. The worst air pollution disaster of modern times struck in London in 1952 when its famous "killer smog" increased the number of deaths in London to 1,600 more than would have normally occurred. Both of those episodes occurred when, under conditions lasting for several days, unusual weather prevented the dispersal of pollutants.

Such major disasters are cause for concern. However, of much greater significance for the American population are the subtle, long-range effects on human health of exposure to low-level, long-lasting pollution.

The causes of chronic diseases which constitute the major public health problems of our time are difficult to determine. Assessing the contribution of particular pollutants to these conditions is complicated by the seemingly infinite variety of pollutants to which persons, particularly those in urban areas, are exposed from the day of their birth. And it is difficult to separate pollution from the other biological and physical stresses to which people are subjected.

Nonetheless, it is well established that air pollution contributes to the incidence of such chronic diseases as emphysema, bronchitis, and other respiratory ailments. Polluted air is also linked to higher mortality rates from other causes, including cancer and arteriosclerotic heart disease. Smokers living in polluted cities have a much higher rate of lung cancer than smokers in rural areas.

The incidence of chronic diseases has soared sharply during this century, while the infectious diseases which were the primary public health concern in the past have been brought under control. Heart and blood vessel diseases caused more than half the deaths in the United States in 1962. Lung cancer, once a rarity, now kills more persons than all other cancer types combined. Emphysema has doubled every 5 years since World War II. Air pollution has been linked to asthma, acute respiratory infections, allergies, and other ailments in children. Such childhood diseases may well underlie chronic ills developed in later life.

Knowledge of the health effects of specific contaminants present in the air is far from complete. However, the more overt health effects of several major classes of pollutants are beginning to be defined. Those pollutants are found almost everywhere in the United States.

When *carbon monoxide* is inhaled, it displaces the oxygen in the blood and reduces the amount carried to the body tissues. At levels commonly found in city air, it can slow the reactions of even the healthiest persons, making them more prone to accidents. Moreover, it is believed to impose an extra burden on those already suffering from anemia, diseases of the heart and blood vessels, chronic lung disease, overactive thyroid, or even simple fever. Cigarette smokers, who are already inhaling significant amounts of CO in tobacco smoke, take on an additional CO burden from polluted air.

Studies show that exposure to 10 parts per million of CO for approximately 8 hours may dull mental performance. Such levels of carbon monoxide are commonly found in cities throughout the world. In heavy traffic situations, levels of 70, 80, or 100 parts per million are not uncommon for short periods.

Sulfur oxides, produced mainly by burning coal and oil, can cause temporary and permanent injury to the respiratory system. When particulate matter is inhaled with the sulfur oxides, health damage increases significantly. The air pollution disasters of recent years were due primarily to sharply increased levels of sulfur oxides and particulates.

Sulfur dioxide can irritate the upper respiratory tract. Carried into the lungs on particles, it can injure delicate tissue. Sulfuric acid—formed from sulfur trioxide when water is present—can penetrate deep into the lungs and damage tissue.

Health may be imperiled when the annual mean concentration of sulfur dioxide in the air rises above 0.04 parts per million. Deaths from bronchitis and from lung cancer may increase when this level of sulfur dioxide is accompanied by smoke concentrations of about 0.06 parts per million. American cities often exceed this annual mean substantially. The annual mean concentration of SO_2 in the air was 0.12 parts per million in Chicago in 1968; in Philadelphia it was 0.08. When SO_x exceeds 0.11 parts per million for 3 to 4 days, adverse health effects have been observed, and this level is reached in many large cities during inversions.

Photochemical oxidants have emerged relatively recently as a major health problem, and research relating to their effects on human health is still in its infancy. However, studies have shown that eye irritation begins when peak oxidant levels reach 0.10 parts per million. Increased frequency of asthma attacks occurs in some patients on those days when hourly concentrations average 0.05 to 0.06 parts per million. Even the healthiest persons may be affected, however; a study of cross-country runners in a Los Angeles high school showed that their performances suffered when hourly average oxidant levels ranged from 0.03 to 0.30 parts per million.

Less is known about the effects on health of *nitrogen oxides,* which play such an important part in producing photochemical pollution. They have been little studied until recently. However, evidence so far suggests that they may be harmful to human health. A study in Chattanooga, Tenn., linked very low levels of these oxides in the air to children's susceptibility to Asian flu.

The lowest *particulate levels* at which health effects have been noted in the United States were reported at Buffalo. The Buffalo study suggests that the overall death rate rises in areas with an annual average concentration ranging from 80 to 100 micrograms per cubic meter. The study also reveals a tie between these levels of particulate matter and gastric cancer in men 50 to 69 years old. A similar association was found in a Nashville study. Particulate levels in this range are found in most major urban areas and are common even in smaller industrial cities.

The findings relating to particulate matter, as a class of pollutants, amply justify measures to reduce their level in the air. Included in this class of pollutants are a number of substances which are potential health hazards at much lower concentrations and which will require even more stringent controls.

Beryllium, for example, which may be emitted from industrial sources and from rocket fuel, can cause lesions in the lung, producing serious respiratory damage and even death. Since the sources of this pollutant are limited, however, it may be a problem only in specific localities.

Asbestos, long recognized as an occupational hazard, is increasingly present in the ambient air because of its use in construction materials, brake linings, and other products. Long exposure in industry produces the lung-scarring disease, asbestosis. On the other hand, mesothelioma, a type of lung cancer associated almost exclusively with asbestos exposure, does not appear to be associated only with heavy or continued exposure.

Many other particulate pollutants are a growing public health worry even though they may not constitute such an immediate and direct threat. Current studies suggest that lead levels now found in the blood and urine of urban populations—although well below those associated with classic lead poisoning—may interfere with the ability of the human body to produce blood. As air pollution becomes more widespread, increased numbers of people are being exposed to airborne lead, chiefly from automotive emissions, at levels formerly found only in congested areas.

. . . to Vegetation and Materials

Air pollution inflicts widespread and costly damage on plant life and buildings and materials. Some experiences of the past warned of the effects of air pollution on plant life. Sulfur dioxide fumes from a large copper smelting plant set up after the Civil War in Copper Basin, Tenn., damaged 30,000 acres of timberland. Much of this originally forested mountain land is still barren. Today, the damage to plant life is less dramatic than in the days of unrestricted smelter operations. But the slower, chronic injury inflicted on agricultural, forest, and ornamental vegetation by increasing quantities and varieties of air pollutants has now spread to all parts of the country.

Smog in the Los Angeles basin contributes to the slow decline of citrus groves south of the city and damages trees in the San Bernardino National Forest

50 miles away. Fluroide and sulfur oxides, released into the air by phosphate fertilizer processing in Florida, have blighted large numbers of pines and citrus orchards. Livestock grazing on fluoride-tainted vegetation develop a crippling condition known as fluorosis. In New Jersey, pollution injury to vegetation has been observed in every country and damage reported to at least 36 commercial crops.

At sulfur oxide levels routinely observed in some of our cities, many plants suffer a chronic injury described as "early aging." Nitrogen dioxide produces similar injury symptoms and seems to restrict the growth of plants even when symptoms of injury are not visible. Ozone, a major photochemical oxidant, is a significant threat to leafy vegetables, field and forage crops, shrubs, and fruit and forest trees—particularly conifers. The damage from ozone in minute quantities can be great. Extended ozone exposure to 0.05 parts per million can reduce a radish yield 50 percent. Tobacco is sensitive to ozone at a level of 0.03 parts per million.

Air pollutants also damage a wide variety of materials. Sulfur oxides will destroy even the most durable products. Steel corrodes two to four times faster in urban industrial areas than it does in rural areas where much less sulfur-bearing coal oil are burned. When particulate matter is also present in the air, the corrosion rates multiply. One-third of the replacement cost of steel rails in England is estimated to be caused by sulfur pollution. The rise of sulfur oxides levels in the air is accelerating the erosion of statuary and buildings throughout the world, and in some cities, works of art made of stone, bronze, and steel must be moved indoors to preserve them from deterioration. Particulate matter in the air not only speeds the corrosive action of other pollutants but by itself is responsible for costly damage and soiling. Clothes and cars must be washed, houses painted, and buildings cleaned more often because of the particulates in the air. Ozone damages textiles, discolors dyes, and greatly accelerates the cracking of rubber.

. . . to Visibility

Air pollution dims visibility, obscures city skylines and scenic beauty, interferes with the safe operation of aircraft and automobiles, and disrupts transportation schedules. In one recent year, low visibility from smoke, haze, and dust was the suspected cause of 15 to 20 plane crashes. In Los Angeles, visibility in the smog frequently lowers to less than 3 miles. During the air pollution alert in the eastern States during July 1970, visibility was almost totally obscured in some areas. The Federal Aviation Administration's visibility safety factor for airplane operation without instruments is 5 miles. Nitrogen dioxide, which reaches peak levels during morning rush-hour traffic, is responsible for the whiskey-brown haze that stains the sky over many cities. Particulates, however, are the major villain in reducing visibility. Particles (ash, carbon, dust, and liquid particles) discharged directly to the air scatter and absorb light, reducing the contrast between objects and their backgrounds. Particles are also formed in the atmosphere by photochemical reactions and by the conversion of sulfur dioxide to sulfuric acid mist. Wherever sulfur pollution is significant—which is wherever large amounts of coal and oil are burned—visibility diminishes as relative humidity rises.

... to Climate

Air pollution alters climate and may produce global changes in temperature.

WHAT AIR POLLUTION COSTS

... in Damages

The total costs of air pollution in the United States cannot be precisely calculated, but they amount to many billions of dollars a year. Economic studies are beginning to identify some of the more obvious costs. To paint steel structures damaged by air pollution runs an estimated $100 million a year. Commercial laundering, cleaning, and dyeing of fabrics soiled by air pollution costs about $800 million. Washing cars dirtied by air pollution costs about $240 million. Damage to agricultural crops and livestock is put at $500 million a year or more. Adverse effects of air pollution on air travel cost from $40 to $80 million a year. Even more difficult to tie down are the costs of replacing and protecting precision instruments or maintaining cleanliness in the production of foods, beverages, and other consumables. It is equally difficult to assess damage, soiling, and added maintenance to homes and furnishings or how air pollution acts on property values. The cost of fuels wasted in incomplete combustion and of valuable and potentially recoverable resources such as sulfur wasted into the air is also hard to count. It is still more difficult to determine the dollar value of medical costs and time lost from work because of air pollution—or to calculate the resulting fall in productivity of business and industry.

... in Control

The total investment necessary through 1975 to control the major industrial and municipal sources of particulate matter, sulfur oxides, hydrocarbons, and carbon monoxide in 100 metropolitan areas of the United States has been estimated at $2.6 billion. This includes costs for controlling both existing and new sources. By 1975, it will cost another $1.9 billion for operation, maintenance, depreciation, and interest.

These estimated costs are based on assumed future control requirements.

Still, the yearly cost to control the industrial sources of these four major pollutants is relatively low, less than 1 percent of the value of the annual output of the industries involved, although the costs to some industries is much greater.

The Health Effects of Air Pollution

What happens inside a man's body when he breathes in, along with his vital oxygen, all the toxic gases and noxious particles that so persistently accompany it in urban life? Scientists have been pressing hard for many years to find out, but the answer is not a simple one. In fact, amassing the necessary knowledge is as complex a project as pollution is a problem.

Information is accumulating, however. This chapter looks at some of what has been learned and describes the methods used to acquire the knowledge. It discusses the respiratory diseases linked to air pollution and examines the links themselves. And it touches on the possible connections between air pollution and nonrespiratory diseases.

THE DIFFICULTY OF FINDING ANSWERS

Some of the ill effects of air pollution have long been public knowledge. Pedestrians knowingly curse the smog as they wipe the tears from their burning eyes. Auto drivers hopefully roll up their windows when traffic fumes threaten to suffocate them. Asthmatics fearfully expect an attack when an inversion sets in.

And, from time to time, the ill effects become headlines, as in Donora, Pennsylvania, in 1948, when almost half the inhabitants were sickened. But even in disasters, the culprit is hard to pin down. Most of the people who sickened or died were already ill. It has been difficult indeed to determine whether air pollution does any lasting damage to healthy people. Or if, in the customary little doses, it does much damage to anyone at all—even to the people with heart or lung diseases who are known to be vulnerable.

To define the ill effects of air pollution, scientists would like to know what substances in the air are harmful and in what way, in what concentrations and combinations, at what times of day or season, at what length of exposure, and for which groups of people.

Yet even the basic testing of a sample of air has its difficulties. For the

Reprinted by permission from *Air Pollution Primer,* National Tuberculosis and Respiratory Disease Association, 1969.

sample cannot be exactly the same as one taken from the next block, from a hundred feet higher, or at a different time of the day or year.

And the constantly changing air is inhaled by different people—old, young, well, sick, tense, or underfed; people with different jobs, from traffic officers who work outdoors to executives who step from air-conditioned car to air-conditioned office.

Other complicating factors are inherent in chemical reactions. Synergism, for example. *Synergism* is the far greater reaction of the body to a combination of chemicals than the total reaction expected from the chemicals acting independently. The effect on the lungs of sulfur dioxide carried on a benzpyrene aerosol is a synergistic one. And the effect of cigarette smoking and air pollution together may be another.

There may also be a *subtractive process.* One pollutant chemical may cancel out another, thereby reducing the effect each may have had alone. Such a process may account for negative reactions in situations where positive ones were expected. For example, small amounts of sulfur dioxide in the air appear to lessen the effects of oxidant on plants.

The possibility also exists of body-built resistance to long-term pollution. One study of people who were regularly exposed to sulfur dioxide in the course of their work, for example, indicated that they experienced little or no irritation of the respiratory tract. (Another study, on the other hand, associated repeated exposure with increased sensitivity.)

Despite all the uncertainties and variables, a great deal has been learned. And, although no simple cause-and-effect relationship has been found between, say, sulfur dioxide and emphysema, evidence piles up, and understanding of the effects of air pollutants on the health of human beings slowly widens and becomes more convincing.

RESEARCH METHODS

Several sources for evidence are available to the scientists: retrospective examination of industrial accidents and acute air pollution episodes, epidemiological and clinical studies—often hand in hand—and controlled laboratory investigations. But none of these methods, alone, can offer clear-cut answers. Let's see why.

Epidemiological Surveys. *Epidemiology* deals with the study of a disease as it affects a community rather than an individual. It concerns itself with the distribution and incidence of the disease; mortality and morbidity rates; and the relationship of climate, age, sex, race, and other factors.

Epidemiological surveys can be—and have been—used to measure the relatively long-term effects of living in an area subject to air pollution. They are valuable because they are concerned with real people exposed to the variety and complexity of a real environment. But, even if carefully planned, epidemiological surveys are limited by precisely that reality. The health of an individual, after all, responds to many things. Some are the variables of the environment, such as weather, industry, and traffic; others are peculiar to him, such as his occupation, age, sex, and smoking habits. (Cigarette smoking is so important a factor in chronic respiratory disease that it may becloud or even conceal the effects of polluted air.)

Epidemiological studies alone, therefore, cannot prove a cause-and-effect relationship. An association can be inferred, however, between a given exposure and a given effect, and the inference can be backed up with corroborating facts established by other methods.

Clinical Studies. Some investigations concern themselves with the disease process in the living subject. They are known as *clinical studies* and can provide backing for epidemiological surmises. Clinical studies can be especially valuable today because of precise pulmonary function measurement techniques. With the aid of such special methods, careful observations of patients can add immensely to the general impressions of the effects of pollution.

Industrial Research. The requirements of industrial hygiene have also provided data that, in the past, had a strong influence on our judgment of what chemicals were harmful. But exposure criteria based on industry's knowledge may be neither adequate nor pertinent. Much of what was discovered was based on studies made only on healthy adult males, using chemicals rarely found in the average atmosphere in the tested form or concentration. (Industrial accidents, however, did give us enough information to warrant caution in new uses of known poisons.)

Laboratory Experiments. Laboratory experiments, too, illuminate potentially damaging processes. True, they are limited because the subjects are not human and the situation is unreal. But they do allow experimentation with what may be dangerous contaminants found in various real situations. And such investigations can support the theory of a relationship between air pollution and disease and demonstrate the complexity of that relationship.

Accidents. Finally, lessons are learned from accidents. Industrial accidents have supplied us, willy-nilly, with much proof of the danger of polluted air. One such accident took place in Poza Rica, Mexico. There, one morning in November, 1950, an accident at the sulfur-producing factory spilled hydrogen sulfide into the atmosphere during a fog-patched inversion. The lesson was swift and impressive: Within a half-hour enough hydrogen sulfide escaped and remained in the air to kill 22 people and cause 320 to be hospitalized.

Other accidents are even more infamous—and more educational. These are the disasters in which, under certain weather conditions, air pollution caused by the ordinary activities of an industrialized area quite clearly brought illness and death to large numbers of people. But these acute episodes, too, have their shortcomings as teaching devices.

Their lessons are not applicable on a wholesale basis, since they are rare occurrences and pollution is a daily menace. Besides, the majority of them occurred before science was prepared to assess them accurately by the sophisticated techniques now available.

Epidemiological and clinical studies, laboratory experiments, industrial research, and accidents—these are the parts of knowledge. Even put together, however, these pieces of information may not be proof positive of direct cause-and-effect relationship. For methods differ from study to study, each trying to test its own hypothesis, and, as a result, proof tends to spread out rather than pile up cumulatively.

The conclusions that follow, nevertheless, are generally accepted and are based on the totality of today's knowledge. Let's look, then, at what we know. It is impressive.

THE ACUTE EPISODES

It was probably the shock of the notorious air pollution disasters, which swept in a wave of acute illnesses and sudden deaths, that first stripped the smokestack of its glory. And turned what was a monument to progress into a gravestone for the dead.

Meuse River Valley, Belgium. The first of the tragedies to arouse worldwide concern occurred in Belgium, in the Meuse River Valley, where a heavily industrialized area extends for some 15 miles. The terrain has a valley topography, typically lending itself to inversions. In retrospect, it is no surprise that the Meuse Valley suffered exceedingly when all of Belgium was blanketed by a thick, cold fog in the first week of December, 1930. Trapped by the inversion, the pollutants gathered day after day and stagnated. Within a few days, thousands fell ill; 60 persons died from the poisoned air. The dead were mostly the elderly and those already very ill from diseases of the heart or lungs. Those who merely sickened complained quickly of coughing and shortness of breath.

Donora, Pennsylvania. Donora was the victim of a similar situation. The town, crammed with industry, is located in the Monongahela River Valley. In October, 1948, during an inversion that covered a wide area of the northeastern United States, Donora had its tragedy. Among a population of only 14,000, close to 6,000 fell ill. Instead of the normal 2 deaths for the period, the fog and pollutant-filled inversion produced 20.

Again, the elderly were hit harder and oftener; again, existing heart or lung disease was a frequent concomitant; and again, most people coughed—although they also suffered from sore throats, chest constriction, headaches, breathlessness, burning and tearing eyes, running nose, vomiting, and nausea.

London, England. The fogs of London are notorious. So is the pollution. For centuries Londoners heated their homes with soft coal in open fireplaces. The resultant smoke and fog—the old original "smog"—combined with the modern contaminants of an industrial city to leave their mark on its inhabitants during a 5-day inversion in December, 1952. This time the deaths of 4,000 people were chalked up to the noxious air.

Give that special London air credit for sickening people, too. More than twice as many as usual. The normal number of weekly applications for emergency bed service in December in London is about 1,000, but during the 1952 episode the weekly number was more than 2,500. Nor did the number of applications subside to normal for 2 to 3 weeks afterwards.

And once more, both illness and death struck oftener at those with pre-existing heart and lung conditions.

London has had other incidents: Six had been recorded earlier, as far back as 1873, with deaths attributed to them totaling over 2,500. It is possible, furthermore, that only the precautions brought about by these earlier calamities kept mortality figures down in a similar inversion in December, 1962. At that time the deaths of a mere 750 people were laid at the door of polluted air.

New York City. Meuse Valley, Donora, London—these were the great and, we hope, bygone disasters. But other areas doubtless harbor their unnoted tragedies, awaiting only the probing eyes of the epidemiologists.

New York City has such probers. According to them, air pollution episodes took place in 1953, 1962, 1963, and 1966. By comparing mortality figures over a number of years, the probers concluded that in 1963, for example, during a period of heavy air pollution, Asian flu, and extreme cold, 405 people died because of air pollution alone. And in 1966, a 3-day period of inversion with air pollution caused the deaths of 168 people. What's more, the fatalities in the 1966 episode were probably much lower than they might have been because the inversion occurred during a Thanksgiving weekend, when many pollution-producing activities were not carried on, and because certain air pollution restrictions were imposed by the city.

THE LESSONS OF THE DISASTERS

Almost immediately after the Meuse Valley incident, investigators drew several conclusions that 30-some years and numerous additional tragedies have corroborated.

The conclusions: (1) The effects of the incidents were anatomically localized and limited to the respiratory tract. (2) The people most vulnerable were those who were elderly and those with pre-existing disease of the cardiorespiratory system. (3) Meteorological conditions were an important factor. (4) Not one but two or more interacting pollutants were responsible—sulfur dioxide, sulfur trioxide, particulate solids, and droplets of fog as carriers.

Using the lessons of the acute episodes, investigators have been trying to flush out their evildoer. In their efforts to identify the villain, scientists have pored over records and statistics. They have mapped the breathing of well people and sick people and animals. They have stuck needles into hamsters, sprayed bacteria at mice, and filled guinea pigs with polluted air. What have they learned?

HOW AIR POLLUTION MAY AFFECT
THE RESPIRATORY TRACT

Air pollution's major effect on health appears to be the result of irritant materials acting on the respiratory tract. The most culpable substances in the matter, it is believed, are the sulfur oxides (with and without particulates), nitrogen dioxide, and ozone and other oxidants.

Sulfur dioxide is relatively soluble in water and dissolves rapidly in the mucus of the upper airways. (*Mucus* is the sticky liquid that covers the airway linings.) Nitrogen dioxide and ozone are less soluble and travel farther. And aerosols of metallic sulfur compounds can be inhaled deeply into the lungs.

Laboratory studies lead to the belief that air pollution may actually alter the body's responses to infectious disease. Over the years a number of different kinds of animals and animal tissues have been exposed to various irritants common in polluted air. The results indicate that both the structure and the function of the respiratory tract may be changed by them.

The many studies suggest these conclusions:

- Certain irritants, either gaseous or particulate, can slow down and even stop the action of the cilia and thus leave the sensitive underlying cells without protection. (The *cilia* are hair-like cells that line the airways. By their sweeping movement they propel the mucus—and the germs and dirt caught in it—out of the respiratory tract.)
- The irritants can cause the production of increased or thickened mucus.
- They can cause a constriction of the airways.
- They can induce swelling or excessive growth of the cells that form the lining of the airways.
- They can cause a loss of cilia or even of several layers of cells.
- Because of one or more of these reactions, breathing may become more difficult, and foreign matter, including bacteria and other micro-organisms, may not be effectively removed, so that respiratory infection can more easily result.

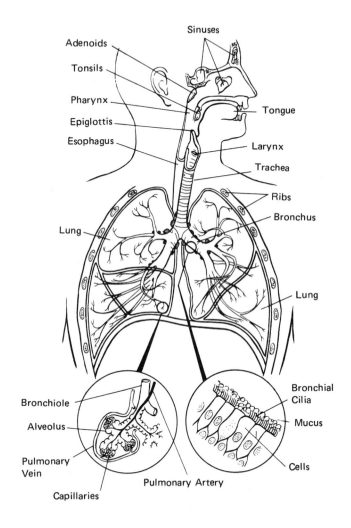

THE RESPIRATORY SYSTEM

SURVEYS LINK POLLUTION TO RESPIRATORY DISEASE

Epidemiological studies present a good case for a link between slow and steady air pollution and respiratory disease, both *chronic* (long-continued) and *acute* (short and relatively severe). A 12-year survey, ending in 1960, of deaths in and around Nashville, Tennessee, indicated that levels of air pollution there were reflected in the death rates from respiratory disease. A study of 38,207 deaths, adjusted for differences in income and social status, revealed that more deaths from breathing ailments occurred in the sections of the city subjected to the heaviest air pollution.

Another study of the inhabitants of two Pennsylvania villages, Seward and New Florence, each with a population of about 1,000, also demonstrates a link between respiratory diseases, both chronic and acute, and air pollution. The two villages were quite similar except that Seward was subject to much higher levels of pollution than New Florence. Those inhabitants of both towns who were 30 years of age or over were given pulmonary function tests, X-rays, and questionnaires on their medical history. The people tested in Seward, the town with heavy pollution, lapsed more often from what the investigators considered normal good health than those tested in New Florence.

Still another survey looked for and found a connection between chronic and acute respiratory disorders and pollution. This one examined hospital admissions in Los Angeles for 223 consecutive days in 1961. The admission records showed a close correlation between high levels of various air pollutants and allergic disorders, acute upper respiratory infections, influenza, bronchitis, and heart, vascular, and respiratory diseases.

ACUTE RESPIRATORY DISEASES

Let's look more carefully now at acute respiratory diseases. The connection has been noted in a number of epidemiological studies. One of them was concerned with the daily ailments of 1,090 New York City adults who lived in a half-square-mile area and who did *not* suffer from chronic cough. The study found that, when they did cough, their coughing was connected with levels of sulfur dioxide and particulate matter in the city air. The coughing did not always result at once, but within a month following a high pollution period, many of the subjects reported that they had developed a cough.

Nonspecific Upper Respiratory Disease. Though the common cold is generally believed to be caused by any of a group of viruses, irritant air pollution appears either to increase one's susceptibiltity to them or at least to produce cold symptoms. These symptoms are medically described as *acute nonspecific upper respiratory disease.*

In the classical episodes—in Donora, Meuse Valley, and London—those who were mildly or moderately affected displayed the symptoms of the common cold.

In a 1950 study in Cumberland, Maryland, interviews showed that there were significantly more common colds among those living in the more heavily polluted section of town.

Another study—a large-scale, continuing survey of absenteeism in industrial plants in several locations in the United States—found that high levels of sulfur oxides and solid particles correlate with increased frequency not only of colds but also of other acute upper respiratory infections.

And investigations in Great Britain, Japan, and the Soviet Union confirm that common colds and other upper respiratory infections occur more often in areas with high pollution levels.

Other Acute Respiratory Diseases. Laboratory investigations have indicated the possible connection of air pollution with deeper, more severe lung disease. Experiments have repeatedly shown that animals forced to inhale some of the irritating gases commonly found in community atmosphere are more vulnerable to pneumonia than animals not exposed to the gaseous irritants. For instance, nitrogen oxides at levels found in urban air pollution do not appear to be directly harmful. Yet after certain strains of mice were exposed to nitrogen oxide in concentrations recorded in Los Angeles, the mice showed an increased mortality from pneumonia.

Experiments with ozone showed a similar significant increase in animals' susceptibility to pneumonia. A laboratory accident also demonstrated a relationship between pollutants and respiratory infections: Caged laboratory animals were accidently exposed to diluted auto exhaust gas. They developed lung infections. Animals housed next to them under identical conditions, except for the accidental gassing, developed no such infections.

This does not imply that the pollutants *caused* the infections. All living things harbor assorted viruses and bacteria; when the body's defenses are weakened, the germs cause active illness. The weakening of these defenses appears to be the role of some air contaminants.

CHRONIC RESPIRATORY DISEASES

Evidence for a connection between air pollution and chronic respiratory disease has also been collected. In addition to the mortality and morbidity figures already cited, there is a noteworthy smaller study of Erie County, New York. Among white men from the ages of 50 to 69 who died between 1949 and 1961, the number of deaths from chronic respiratory illness—the figure was adjusted for socio-economic influence—was twice as high in areas of high air pollution as in low ones.

The Factor of Chronic Airway Resistance. Polluting irritants in the respiratory tract do more than prepare it for infections. They produce a condition that appears to be a factor in a number of chronic respiratory diseases—a condition known as chronic airway resistance.

Airway resistance is the narrowing of the air passages in response to the presence of irritating substances, thus making breathing difficult. The phenomenon is being seen not only as a temporary constriction but as a permanent effect. In the study of people over 30 in Seward and New Florence, Pennsylvania, investigators found a significant difference in the airway resistance and the lung capacity of the inhabitants of the two towns—a difference that apparently related to the differing amounts of long-term air pollution they were exposed to.

No single pollutant can be named with assurance as the cause of any chronic disease. Experiments, however, point especially to the sulfur oxides as culprits, since they produce immediate airway constriction. And studies with laboratory animals show that when sulfur oxides are carried on aerosols, especially aerosols in a size range found in urban air, the combination of the two elicits the greatest increase in resistance.

Ozone has also been shown to produce a thickening of the bronchiolar walls, at least in some animals. This reaction occurred in a study in which a number of animals of different species inhaled ozone for 400 days at concentrations slightly higher than that common in some urban areas. Other reactions in this study included inflammation of the bronchi and the bronchioles, some injury to the trachea and bronchi, and death from pneumonia for many animals that didn't last through the whole experiment.

A different kind of study was conducted with guinea pigs that had somewhat higher airway resistance to begin with. (They might correspond to people with respiratory disease.) When the guinea pigs and control animals were exposed to an irritant aerosol or gas, the air passages in both groups narrowed, but the guinea pigs developed more resistance than the controls did.

Bronchial Asthma. Asthma is a kind of airway resistance, too, of course, although air pollution cannot take all the credit for it.

Bronchial asthma is caused by an allergy. It is a state of abnormal responsiveness of the air passages to certain substances. An attack consists of a widespread narrowing of the smaller airways—the bronchioles—by a muscle spasm, a swelling of the mucous membrane, or a thickening and increase of mucous secretions. But, even though chronic, the condition is temporary. Without a complicating disease, the bronchioles return to a normal state after an attack.

Physicians can recite long lists of stimuli capable of triggering asthma attacks. On those lists, at least for some people, is polluted air, for man-made community air pollution has been known to bring an asthma or asthma-like attacks. (Sulfur dioxide has been cited as one of the many specific producers of allergic reactions in asthma sufferers.)

Clearly related to air pollution, though not so clearly definable as asthma, is what is usually referred to as Tokyo-Yokohama asthma. This disease became known in 1946, when it reached epidemic proportions in Yokohama—a highly

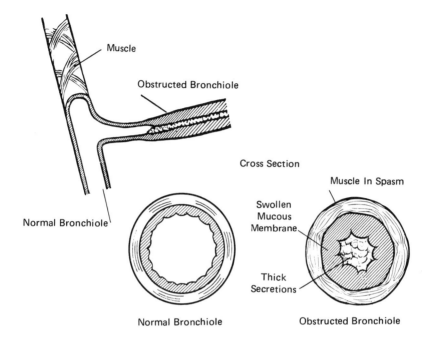

BRONCHIAL ASTHMA

Two views of a bronchiole, showing how it may be obstructed during an asthma attack.

industrialized city. The disease first appeared among American troops stationed there and then spread to their dependents living in the area. Later the same condition was found among our military personnel in the Tokyo area. In both places, there appeared to be an obvious relationship between the asthmatic attacks and the levels of air pollution. But the illness differed from true asthma in that most of those afficted had no history of allergy, and, when the afflicted left the area, especially if their stays were short, they usually had no further attacks.

Physicians are loath to call the condition asthma under these circumstances; the diagnosis of asthmatic bronchitis is more readily accepted. Whatever the label attached to it, the disease appears to be a reality. Studies conducted in 1960 in a pulmonary function laboratory revealed that, despite the vanished symptoms, the effects lingered. Further studies in 1962 on 244 patients who returned to the United States showed that two-thirds of them still had abnormal breathing patterns. In some, too, emphysema had developed. But almost all the 620 patients diagnosed as having Tokyo-Yokohama asthma were moderate-to-heavy smokers.

This country has its own problems. Pasadena, California, and Nashville, Tennessee, have both seen asthmatics suffer attacks that seem to be brought on by air pollution.

Even better known, perhaps, for its epidemic outbreaks of asthma is New Orleans. A number of studies have been undertaken to discover the source of the attacks. Possible links have been suggested between the asthma outbreaks and different sources, among them a grain elevator and a city dump. And even though the source is not positively identified, the link to air pollution seems clear. A study of daily admission rates for asthmatic emergencies in one hospital between 1953 and 1960 showed that rates leaped from the usual 25 or so to 200 when a gentle southwest wind prevailed. During a single week in October, 1962, more than 300 asthmatics sought treatment, and 9 asthmatic patients died.

Chronic Bronchitis. What we know about chronic bronchitis and its relationship to air pollution is muddied by disagreements over definition. In this country a diagnosis of *chronic bronchitis* is considered justified when an excessive amount of mucus is produced in the bronchi and a lasting or recurrent cough results and other diseases that cause such a cough—such as lung infections, tumors, or heart disease—are absent. (Chest specialists set an arbitrary minimum for the cough of 3 months a year for at least 2 successive years.)

The British have different standards for the diagnosis of chronic bronchitis. These differences may be at least partially responsible for the proportionately higher number of chronic bronchitis patients recorded in their country. Whatever the reasons, the prevalence of the ailment there has occasioned a great many studies of it. And in Great Britain air pollution—like cigarette smoking—is considered to be a distinct cause of chronic bronchitis.

Statistical associations of chronic bronchitis death rates with air pollution have been demonstrated in Great Britain. In clinical studies of the illness, too, the connection is consistent: Persons suffering from chronic bronchitis, kept under regular observation, show worsening symptoms on days when air pollution levels are high.

Here are some examples of the information the British have collected:

- A 3-year study of men over 45 in a number of county boroughs of England and Wales showed a significant correlation between death rates from chronic bronchitis and sulfur dioxide concentrations.

- A 6-year study of British postmen showed them to be absent from work more often because of chronic bronchitis when they worked outdoors in polluted areas. In the areas of heaviest pollution there were 3 times as many absences as in low-pollution areas.

- A 5-year study of 53 county and metropolitan boroughs of England, Scotland, and Wales showed a highly significant correlation between bronchitis and the amount of acid in rain or snow (acidity that might be caused by sulfur oxide's mixing with droplets of moisture to form sulfuric acid).

In this country information on chronic bronchitis is less easily come by. Americans have been studying the disease for less time, for one thing. And cigarette smoking appears to be so overwhelmingly significant that investigators are having a hard time identifying the role of air pollution.

The disease is growing here, in any case. In the 10 years ending with 1961, the death rate from chronic bronchitis increased 50 per cent, and approximately the same increase occurred in the five years following. Nor does the 1966 figure of 4,412 deaths caused by chronic bronchitis present an accurate picture. A recent study concluded that the reported death rate for chronic bronchitis and emphysema is low by from 25 to 50 per cent. These diseases are listed more often as a contributing cause than as the primary cause of death.

One investigation here—using as its criterion a chronic cough that brings up phlegm (mucus) on most days for three months of two successive years—found chronic bronchitis in 21 per cent of a series of men 40 to 59 years of age.

The irritation of the bronchial tubes that causes the chronic bronchitis coughing is abetted by recurrent acute bronchial infections. And, at least in mice, the two major defenses of the bronchi against infection—the flow of mucus and the ability of cells to destroy bacteria—appear to be diminished or stopped by the inhalation of polluted air, thereby allowing bacteria to reach the usually sterile bronchial tree. Clinical studies of bronchitis patients, furthermore, indicate that bacterial infection within the bronchi causes lingering damage. Bacteria remain there, and the bronchi are more susceptible to infection in the future.

Pulmonary Emphysema. Closely linked to chronic bronchitis is pulmonary emphysema. Indeed, emphysema may be its follow-up as well as its companion.

Emphysema is an anatomic change in the lungs that shows itself in shortness of breath. It is characterized by a breakdown of the walls of the *alveoli,* the tiny air spaces beyond the terminal bronchioles. (The *bronchioles* are the smaller branches of the bronchial tree.) As the disease progresses, the alveoli become enlarged, lose their resilience, and their walls disintegrate—irreversible tissue changes.

No single factor can be said to be the original cause of emphysema. Asthma and chronic bronchitis are often found in the patient with emphysema; both can increase the severity of the disease. The symptoms of all these diseases are aggravated by air pollution. What is known of the action of air-polluting irritants on the respiratory system in general, therefore, justifies the search for a causal connection between air pollution and emphysema.

Because this disease has so recently gained national attention, little work has yet been done to determine the possibility or strength of the association between it and polluted air. One recent study, however, certainly indicates that a strong relationship exists. (The relationship is even stronger when cigarette smoking is a factor.) This is a study of autopsies of the lungs of 300 inhabitants of heavily polluted St. Louis and an equal number from relatively unpolluted

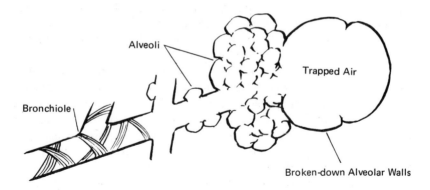

Alveoli

Trapped Air

Bronchiole

Broken-down Alveolar Walls

PULMONARY EMPHYSEMA

The loss of elasticity and the deterioration of the alveoli walls deters the exhalation of carbon dioxide.

Winnipeg, Canada. Investigators found 4 times as much severe emphysema among cigarette smokers in St. Louis as among smokers in Winnipeg. And even among nonsmokers, in whose lungs no severe emphysema existed, there was 3 times as much mild to moderate emphysema among St. Louis inhabitants as among those from Winnipeg. In general, the investigators concluded, emphysema appeared to be more prevalent in St. Louis than Winnipeg, to develop much earlier, and to progress more rapidly.

There are other signs of a connection between emphysema and air pollution. Emphysema is the fastest growing cause of death in the United States. The 20,252 deaths from it in 1966 reflect a 17-fold increase since 1950. And, as with respiratory disease in general, the urban death rate is significantly higher than the rural one—about twice as high, in fact.

In recent years, an average of more than 1,000 workers a month have been forced to retire prematurely because of emphysema. Over 6 per cent of those who receive monthly Social Security disability payments suffer from it—a percentage exceeded only by those with arteriosclerotic heart disease. A recent review of the case histories of more than 50,000 emphysema patients indicates that air pollution could have been a factor in their illness, although cigarette smoking was of far greater importance.

We also know that people with emphysema—and other chronic respiratory diseases—feel worse during periods of severe air pollution. A clinical study of emphysema patients, for example, showed that they felt better and were able to breathe more easily after they were removed from Los Angeles smog and placed in a purified atmosphere for 24 hours.

Lung Cancer. *Lung cancer* is characterized by an abnormal, disorderly new cell growth originating in the bronchial mucous membrane. It is usually fatal.

Lung cancer, like emphysema, cannot be attributed to any single cause. But it seems very likely that atmospheric contaminants, together with other factors—especially cigarette smoking—contribute to the development of this disease.

Agents that produce cancer in laboratory animals have been found wherever they have been sought in polluted city air. Many scientists believe, further, that those atmospheric pollutants which paralyze ciliary action in the respiratory tract may play a role in the development of cancer, even though they are not carcinogens themselves. The paralysis of the cilia would permit cancer-causing substances to remain in contact with the sensitive bronchial cells over a long period of time.

Mortality statistics are persuasive, Deaths from cancer of the lungs, especially among males, have been increasing rapidly in recent years. In the largest metropolitan areas in the United States, the death rate is twice that of rural sections. Significantly, the rate is generally in direct proportion to city population size, as, in general, is the degree of air pollution. Even when cancer death rates are adjusted to take smoking habits and age into consideration, they are still a third higher in large cities than in rural areas.

Many epidemiological studies contribute to the theorized relationship.

- A 1956 report showed that British immigrants to New Zealand had a higher incidence of lung cancer than New Zealand-born persons of the same stock. Britain has far more pollution than New Zealand, and those who lived part of their lives in Britain would naturally have been exposed to more pollution than people born and raised in New Zealand.
- A 1959 study indicated that deaths due to lung cancer among 45- to 64-year-old male British immigrants to South Africa (South Africa too, has less air pollution than Britain) were 44 per cent higher than among native-born South Africans of the same sex and age range—this in spite of the fact that South Africans have long been considered the world's heaviest cigarette smokers.
- Still another epidemiological study showed that the incidence of lung cancer varied with the amount of air pollution: Among Norwegians living in Norway, where the air pollution is low, the lung cancer rate was low. Among Americans living in America, where air pollution is heavy, the rate was twice as high. Among Norwegians who migrated to the United States, the rate was halfway between.

In all these studies, the conclusion was that the contrast in cancer incidence between countries could be laid at the door of air pollution.

The rising incidence of lung cancer has been associated with a number of factors. One is influenza. To investigate this hypothesis, researchers infected mice with flu virus. Survivors had only a slightly higher cancer rate than mice used for controls. Then the experiment continued by exposing these same

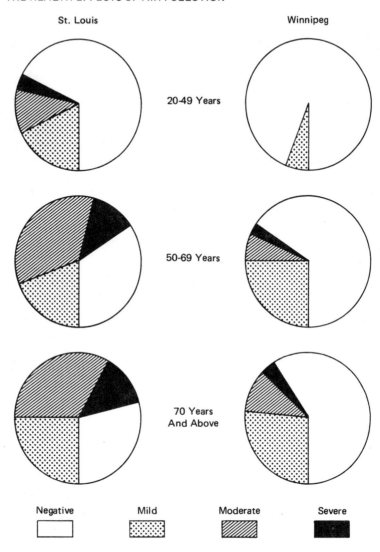

St. Louis

Winnipeg

20-49 Years

50-69 Years

70 Years
And Above

Negative   Mild   Moderate   Severe

**PREVALENCE OF EMPHYSEMA IN TWO CITIES
WITH CONTRASTING LEVELS OF AIR POLLUTION**

Prevalence of emphysema, as found in a 1960-66 post-mortem examination of the lungs of 300 residents of heavily industrialized St. Louis, Missouri and an equal number from relatively unpolluted Winnipeg, Canada. The subjects were well matched by sex, occupation, socio-economic status, length of residence, smoking habits, and age at death. The findings clearly suggest a link between air pollution and pulmonary emphysema.

survivors of the flu to artificial smog (ozonized gasoline)—and the cancer incidence increased manyfold.

Further evidence of pollution's possible role in lung cancer has been unearthed in the laboratory. Mice were painted with carcinogenic hydrocarbons, and tumors resulted. Other mice were exposed to artificially produced photo-chemical smog, and both skin and lung cancers appeared. Mice and rats had certain hydrocarbons implanted in their lungs, and they developed lung cancers. Hamsters had benzpyrene inserted with iron oxide into their tracheas, and they too developed lung cancers. None of these experiments duplicate the conditions in which human beings confront air pollution. But they do demonstrate the potential link between cancer and pollution.

OTHER EFFECTS

The case against air pollution appears to rest heavily upon effects on the respiratory system. But that may be because these are the most obvious effects and, therefore, the first to be investigated. We must also note the testimony of further assaults on human health for which polluted air may be responsible.

Heart disease, for instance. All chronic respiratory disease involves the heart, for stress on the heart and blood vessels is an inevitable result of the constricted or otherwise obstructed and injured respiratory tract. The cardiorespiratory system functions as a unit, one part making up for the occasional failure of the other. The heart must work harder to pump enough blood to compensate for any loss of oxygen due to respiratory disease. As a result, the heart may show significant changes—sometimes doubling in size—as a secondary effect of lung affliction.

The heart's burden is also increased by carbon monoxide, which can reduce the oxygen content of the blood. We don't know how much of a hazard is presented by small quantities of this gas, but such amounts may have a deleterious effect on the hearts of those already suffering from anemia or a cardiorespiratory disease.

Air pollution's effect on the heart was demonstrated during the well-known disasters by the high rates of sickness and death for people with chronic heart disease. The Los Angeles study of hospital admissions mentioned on page 60, correlating high air pollution levels with heart and other disorders, reinforces the conclusion.

And national mortality figures add additional weight: Death rates for coronary heart disease are 37 per cent higher for men and 46 per cent higher for women in metropolitan areas than they are in nonmetropolitan areas. An Illinois study found cardiovascular death rates more than 25 per cent higher for male Chicagoans between 25 and 34 years of age than for their counterparts in rural areas; the difference was 100 per cent for men between 35 and 54; and nearly 200 per cent for men between 55 and 64.

Air pollution is implicated in other symptoms, too. The effects of air pollution on the human eye are well known. Burning, tearing eyes are an immediate reaction to both photochemical smog and sulfur dioxide. Three-fourths of the people surveyed in the metropolitan area of southern California said they were affected by eye irritation. The report of 1,090 New York City residents mentioned on page 60 showed that they suffered from such irritation during periods of high pollution. Studies by eye specialists, however, do not indicate any permanent injury, even from repeated irritation.

Dizziness, headaches, blurred vision, and slowed-down responses are well-known laboratory reactions to certain concentrations of carbon monoxide in the air, although these reactions have not been verified in actual atmospheric conditions.

Less obvious effects of air pollution—carrying inferences for human health— are also coming to light through investigations of various sorts.

- An experiment in California showed that long-continued exposure to artificial smog reduced the fertility of parent mice and the survival rate of their newborn.
- Another experiment showed that mice exposed to artificial smog were less active than mice breathing filtered air.
- Still another experiment indicated that chicks exposed to simulated smog began laying eggs at an earlier age than unexposed chicks. Time has yet to tell if this is a sign of premature aging.

Tomorrow, improved techniques of detection and more precise studies will add to what we now know of the role of air pollution on human health. In the meantime, the tocsin rightly tolls.

III. UNDERSTANDING WATER

AND

SOLID WASTE POLLUTION

Water Pollution

INTRODUCTION

Americans generally assume that the water from their faucets is healthful and free of bacterial or chemical contaminants that can cause disease. Usually, the assumption is correct. The drinking water supplies in cities and towns of the United States rank in quality on the average among the best in the world. Nevertheless, there is cause for serious concern. The major findings from a recently completed Public Health Service, "Community Water Supply Study" show that: 36% of 2,600 individual tap water samples contained one or more bacterial or chemical constituents exceeding public health limits; 53% of the systems evidenced physical deficiencies in ground water sources, inadequate disinfection capacity, inadequate clarification capacity, and/or inadequate system pressure; 77% of the water plant operators were inadequately trained in fundamental water microbiology and 46% were deficient in chemistry relating to their plant operation; 79% of the systems were not inspected by state or county authorities in 1968, the last full calendar year prior to the study; and in 50% of the cases, plant officials did not remember when, if ever, a state or local health department had last surveyed the supply. Man must be protected against such physical, chemical and bacteriological health hazards. The most practical means of accomplishing this is through prevention and control of pollutants at their source, rather than by attempting to prevent or control their transmission through water courses, to cleanse water after it is polluted, or to protect potential receptors from coming in contact with polluted water.

Mission

The mission of a water hygiene program is protection of human health through maintenance of water quality. It insures that persons do not suffer acute or chronic disease from drinking water, using recreational waters, or consuming foods grown or processed with water.

Excerpts from *Environmental Health Planning,* U.S. Department of Health, Education and Welfare, Public Health Service Publication 2120, Bureau of Community Environmental Management, 1971.

PROBLEMS

Despite broad acceptance of PHS Drinking Water Standards, based largely on protection from pathogenic organisms, over 6,000 of the Nation's public water supplies (serving 58 million people) do not serve those standards. As a result, disease outbreaks occur too frequently. Unfortunately, local-state-federal reporting and investigative mechanisms are inadequate to catalogue all cases of waterborne disease. Lack of state and local personnel, inadequate laboratory facilities, and untrained and underpaid water plant operators are primary contributing factors. Similarly, there is a need for improved technology in water treatment methods. PHS Drinking Water Standards are the basis for state standards. Some states have adopted them as written, some have adopted them with minor changes, some use them officially and some unofficially. No state has adopted substantially different standards. Careful reading of the Standards reveals that a high level of facility and operation are required to meet them. The surveying engineer modifies requirements as appropriate for each water supply, but the constant reference point is the Standards. While strict compliance with existing criteria and standards provide considerable health protection to the consumer, actual or potential threats to humans, perhaps more acute than those covered by existing standards, are posed by chemical contaminants, many of which pass through present-day waste and water treatment plants essentially unchanged and undiminished. Some of these, such as lead and radioactive chemicals, have cumulative, long-term deleterious effects, including chronic and incapacitating illnesses.

As our Nation grows, there is corresponding growth in the volume and complexity of chemical wastes entering rivers, lakes and underground aquifers. While precise health effects of chemical pollutants are being determined, capability to routinely test for their presence is being implemented, and methodology to remove or exclude them is being developed, the bodies of most Americans will be serving as filters and accumulators for these substances. Increased use of water for recreation and food production has resulted in greater exposure of man to threats to health and well-being because of the unsafe quality of many such waters. Conversely, certain substances found in water may have a beneficial effect on man. Fluoride as a preventive of dental caries is a well-known example. It took approximately 200 years for our population to pass the 200 million mark. Estimates indicate it will take less than 50 years to reach 400 million, and that by 2020 this Nation will have a population of 468 million. In 1965, we used 269,617 million gallons of water per day; by 2020, estimated use will be 1,368,088 million gallons. To help meet projected requirements, numerous federal and state agencies are planning development of water and related land resources to insure that future water needs for domestic, municipal, industrial, agricultural, power and recreational uses are met. This development requires adequate consideration of health aspects including epidemiological assessment and disease vector control, and environmental health analysis. Failure to give adequate consideration to the health aspects during early planning may result in severe and costly health problems in the future. Projections indicate that water reuse will become more common as populations, demands for goods, and water requirements increase. The effect of impurities will be an increasing problem and input of health officials in the long-range planning process will be increasingly important.

Nation-wide problems in the field of water hygiene include:

1. Water quality does not meet existing standard.
2. Facilities not operated in accordance with accepted standards.
3. Inadequate or incomplete standards due to lack of knowledge of the relation between health and certain pollutants and contaminants found in water.
4. Inadequate knowledge and consideration of health aspects in long-term planning and development of water and related-land resources.
5. Inadequate water treatment facilities and trained operators.
6. Inadequate surveillance of contaminants of public water supplies.

State and local problems are primarily those of providing for facilities and operation that meet minimum criteria for health protection. Provision of facilities and hiring of competent operators is usually the responsibility of the water supply utility. The role of environmental health agencies is that of overseer of operation on behalf of the public to insure the continuous availability of potable water and as a catalyst for planning and providing facilities so they will be available when required. The tools are people and laboratories. In addition to people who obtain water from piped, community systems, a certain segment of the population provides its own water supply.

Increasing urbanization is steadily reducing the number of persons served by individual water supplies but the percentage still varies from around 10 to 35, depending on the areas of the country.

The Limited War on Water Pollution

Gene Bylinsky

To judge by the pronouncements from Washington, we can now start looking forward to cleaner rather than ever dirtier rivers. The Administration has declared a "war" on pollution, and Secretary of the Interior Walter J. Hickel says "we do not intend to lose." Adds Murray Stein, enforcement chief of the Federal Water Pollution Control Administration: "I think we are on the verge of a tremendous cleanup."

The nationwide campaign to clean up ravaged rivers and lakes does seem to be moving a bit. For the first time since the federal government got into financing construction of municipal sewage plants in 1956, Congress has come close to providing the kind of funding it had promised. Assuming the Budget Bureau allows Interior to spend all of the $800 million appropriated for the current fiscal year, that will come to almost two-thirds as much as all the federal funds invested in the program so far. There are other signs that the war is intensifying. Under the provisions of the Water Quality Act of 1965 and the Clean Water Restoration Act of 1966, federal and state officials are establishing water-quality standards and plans for their implementation, to be carried out eventually through coordinated federal-state action. Timetables for new municipal and industrial treatment facilities are being set, surveillance programs are being planned, and tougher federal enforcement authority is being formulated. Without waiting for these plans to materialize, Interior is talking tough to some municipal and industrial polluters, with the possibility of court action in the background.

Even with all this, however, the water-pollution outlook is far from reassuring. Although the nation has invested about $15 billion since 1952 in the construction of 7,500 municipal sewage-treatment plants, industrial treatment plants, sewers, and related facilities, a surprising 1,400 communities in the U.S., including good-sized cities like Memphis, and hundreds of industrial plants still dump untreated wastes into the waterways. Other cities process their sewage only superficially, and no fewer than 300,000 industrial plants discharge their used water into municipal sewage plants that are not equipped to process many of the complex new pollutants.

Since the volume of pollutants keeps expanding while water supply stays basically the same, more and more intervention will be required just to keep things from getting worse. Within the next fifty years, according to some forecasts, the country's population will double, and the demand for water by cities, .industries, and agriculture has tended to grow even faster than the population. These water uses now add up to something like 350 billion gallons a day (BGD), but by 1980, by some estimates, they will amount to 600 BGD. By the year 2000, demand for water is expected to reach 1,000 BGD, considerably exceeding the essentially unchanging supply of dependable fresh water, which is estimated at 650 BGD. More and more, water will have to be reused, and it will cost more and more to retrieve clean water from progressively dirtier waterways.

Just how bad water pollution can get was dramatically illustrated last summer when the oily, chocolate-brown Cuyahoga River in Cleveland burst into flames, nearly destroying two railroad bridges. The Cuyahoga is so laden with industrial and municipal wastes that not even the leeches and sludge worms that thrive in many badly polluted rivers are to be found in its lower reaches. Many other U.S. rivers are becoming more and more like that flammable sewer.

Even without human activity to pollute it, a stream is never absolutely pure, because natural pollution is at work in the form of soil erosion, deposition of leaves and animal wastes, solution of minerals, and so forth. Over a long stretch of time, a lake can die a natural death because of such pollution. The natural process of eutrophication, or enrichment with nutrients, encourages the growth of algae and other plants, slowly turning a lake into a bog. Man's activities enormously speed up the process.

TOO MUCH DEMAND FOR OXYGEN

But both lakes and rivers have an impressive ability to purify themselves. Sunlight bleaches out some pollutants. Others settle to the bottom and stay there. Still others are consumed by beneficial bacteria. These bacteria need oxygen, which is therefore vital to self-purification. The oxygen that sustains bacteria as well as fish and other organisms is replenished by natural aeration from the atmosphere and from life processes of aquatic plants.

Trouble starts when demand for dissolved oxygen exceeds the available supply. Large quantities of organic pollutants such as sewage alter the balance. Bacteria feeding upon the pollutants multiply and consume the oxygen. Organic debris accumulates. Anaerobic areas develop, where microorganisms that can live and grow without free oxygen decompose the settled solids. This putrefaction produces foul odors. Species of fish sensitive to oxygen deficiency can no longer survive. Chemical, physical, and biological characteristics of a stream are altered, and its water becomes unusable for many purposes without extensive treatment.

Pollution today is very complex in its composition, and getting more so all the time. In polluted streams and lakes hundreds of different contaminants can be found: bacteria and viruses; pesticides and weed killers; phosphorus from fertilizers, detergents, and municipal sewage; trace amounts of metals; acid from mine drainage; organic and inorganic chemicals, many of which are so new that we do not know their long-term effects on human health; and even traces of drugs. (Steroid drugs such as the Pill, however, are neutralized by bacteria.)

A distinction is often made between industrial and municipal wastes, but it is difficult to sort them out because many industrial plants discharge their wastes into municipal sewer systems. As a result, what is referred to as municipal waste is also to a large extent industrial waste. By one estimate, as much as 40 percent of all waste water treated by municipal sewage plants comes from industry. Industry's contribution to water pollution is sometimes measured in terms of "population equivalent." Pollution from organic industrial wastes analogous to sewage is now said by some specialists to be about equivalent to a population of 210 million.

The quality of waste water is often measured in terms of its biochemical oxygen demand (BOD), or the amount of dissolved oxygen that is needed by bacteria in decomposing the wastes. Waste water with much higher BOD content than sewage is produced by such operations as leather tanning, beet-sugar refining, and meatpacking. But industry also contributes a vast amount of non-degradable, long-lasting pollutants, such as inorganic and synthetic organic chemicals that impair the quality of water. All together, manufacturing activities, transportation, and agriculture probably account for about two-thirds of all water degradation.

Industry also produces an increasingly important pollutant of an entirely different kind—heat. Power generation and some manufacturing processes use great quantities of water for cooling, and it goes back into streams warmer than it came out. Power plants disgorging great masses of hot water can raise the stream temperature by ten or twenty degrees in the immediate vicinity of the plant. Warmer water absorbs less oxygen and this slows down decomposition of organic matter. Fish, being cold-blooded, cannot regulate their body temperatures, and the additional heat upsets their life cycles; for example, fish eggs may hatch too soon. Some scientists have estimated that by 1980 the U.S. will be producing enough waste water and heat to consume, in dry weather, all the oxygen in all twenty-two river basins in the U.S.

DESIGNED FOR A SIMPLER WORLD

How clean do we want our waterways to be? In answering that question we have to recognize that many of our rivers and lakes serve two conflicting purposes—they are used both as sewers and as sources of drinking water for about 100 million Americans. That's why the new water-quality standards for interstate streams now being set in various states generally rely on criteria established by the Public Health Service for sources of public water supplies. In all, the PHS lists no fewer than fifty-one contaminants or characteristics of water supplies that should be controlled. Many other substances in the drinking water are not on the list, because they haven't yet been measured or even identified. "The poor water-treatment plant operator really doesn't know what's in the stream—what he is treating," says James H. McDermott, director of the Bureau of Water Hygiene in the PHS. With more than 500 new or modified chemicals coming on the market every year, it isn't easy for the understaffed PHS bureaus to keep track of new pollutants. Identification and detailed analysis of pollutants is just beginning as a systematic task. Only a few months ago the PHS established its first official committee to evaluate the effects of insecticides on health.

Many water-treatment plants are hopelessly outmoded. They were designed for a simpler, less crowded world. About three-fourths of them do not go beyond disinfecting water with chlorine. That kills bacteria but does practically nothing to remove pesticides, herbicides, or other organic and inorganic chemicals from the water we drink.

A survey by the PHS, still in progress, shows that most waterworks operators lack formal training in treatment processes, disinfection, microbiology, and chemistry. The men are often badly paid. Some of them, in smaller communities, have other full-time jobs and moonlight as water-supply operators. The survey, encompassing eight metropolitan areas from New York City to Riverside, California, plus the State of Vermont, so far has revealed that in seven areas about 9 percent of the water samples indicated bacterial contamination. Pesticides were found in small concentrations in many samples. In some, trace metals exceeded PHS limits. The level of nitrates, which can be fatal to babies, was too high in some samples. Earlier last year the PHS found that nearly sixty communities around the country, including some large cities, could be given only "provisional approval" for the quality of their water-supply systems. Charles C. Johnson Jr., administrator of the Consumer Protection and Environmental Health Service in the PHS, concluded that the U.S. is "rapidly approaching a crisis stage with regard to drinking water" and is courting "serious health hazards."

Clearly, there will have to be enormous improvement in either the treatment of water we drink or the treatment of water we discard (if not both). The second approach would have the great advantage of making our waterways better for swimming and fishing and more aesthetically enjoyable. And it is more rational anyway not to put poisons in the water in the first place. The most sensible way to keep our drinking water safe is to have industry, agriculture, and municipalities stop polluting water with known and potentially hazardous substances.

Some of this could be accomplished by changing manufacturing processes and recycling waste water inside plants. The wastes can sometimes be retrieved at a profit.

SEWAGE ON THE ROCKS

A great deal of industrial and municipal waste water now undergoes some form of treatment. So-called primary treatment is merely mechanical. Large floating objects such as sticks are removed by a screen. The sewage then passes through settling chambers where filth settles to become raw sludge. Primary treatment removes about one-third of gross pollutants. About 30 percent of Americans served by sewers live in communities that provide only this much treatment.

Another 62 percent live in communities that carry treatment a step beyond, subjecting the effluent from primary processing to secondary processing. In this age of exact science, secondary treatment looks very old-fashioned. The effluent flows, or is pumped, onto a "trickling filter," a bed of rocks three to ten feet deep. Bacteria normally occurring in sewage cover the rocks, multiply, and consume most of the organic matter in the waste water. A somewhat more modern version is the activated sludge process, in which sewage from primary settling tanks is pumped to an aeration tank. Here, in a speeded-up imitation of what a stream does naturally, the sewage is mixed with air and sludge saturated with bacteria. It is allowed to remain for a few hours while decomposition takes place. Properly executed secondary treatment will reduce degradable organic waste by 90 percent. Afterward, chlorine is sometimes added to the water to kill up to 99 percent of disease germs.

Secondary treatment in 90 percent of U.S. municipalities within the next five years and its equivalent in most industrial plants is a principal objective of the current war on pollution. The cost will he high: an estimated $10 billion in public funds for municipal treatment plants and sewers and about $3.3 billion of industry's own funds for facilities to treat wastes at industrial plants.

But today that kind of treatment isn't good enough. Widespread use of secondary treatment will cut the amount of gross sewage in the waterways, but will do little to reduce the subtler, more complex pollutants. The effluents will still contain dissolved organic and inorganic contaminants. Among the substances that pass largely unaffected through bacterial treatment are salts, certain dyes, acids, persistent insecticides and herbicides, and many other harmful pollutants.

Technical "tunnel vision," or lack of thinking about all the possible consequences of a process, has often been the curse of twentieth-century science and technology. Today's sewage plants generally do not remove phosphorus and nitrogen from waste water, but turn the organic forms of these nutrients into mineral forms that are *more* usable by algae and other plants. As one scientist has noted, overgrowths of algae and other aquatic plants then rot to "recreate the same problem of oxygen-consuming organic matter that the sewage plant was designed to control in the first place." The multibillion-dollar program to treat waste water in the same old way, he says, is "sheer insanity."

Yet the U.S. has little choice. Most of the advanced treatment techniques are either still experimental or too costly to be introduced widely. To wait for those promising new methods while doing nothing in the meantime could result in a major pollution calamity.

MATS OF ALGAE AND MOUNTAINS OF FOAM

The pollutants that secondary treatment fails to cope with will increase in volume as industry and population grow. Phosphates, for instance, come in large amounts from detergents and fertilizers, and from human wastes. Phosphorus has emerged as a major pollutant only in recent years. Nitrogen, the other key nutrient for algal growth, is very difficult to control because certain blue-green algae can fix nitrogen directly from the air. Since phosphorus is more controllable, its removal from effluents is critically important to limiting the growth of algae.

A few years ago, when it looked as if America's streams and lakes were to become highways of white detergent foam, the manufacturers converted the detergent base from alkyl benzene sulphonate to a much more biologicallly degradable substance, linear alkylate sulphonate. That effectively reduced the amount of foam but did almost nothing to reduce the amount of phosphates in detergents. The mountains of foam have shrunk, but green mats of algae keep on growing. The developers of detergents failed to consider the possible side effects; such lack of systematic thinking and foresight is precisely what has led to today's environmental abuses.

It might be possible to substitute nonphosphorus bases in detergent manufacture—and work is in progress along those lines. There is a bill before Congress that would ban phosphorus from detergents by the middle of 1971. But this certainly wouldn't do much to restore algae-clogged lakes such as Lake Erie, where farms, cities, and factories all contribute phosphates.

There is little prospect of substituting something else for the phosphate in fertilizer. It's hard to visualize a fertilizer that is a nutrient when applied to land and not a nutrient when it enters the water. One way to reduce water pollution from farmlands would be to reduce the amounts of chemical fertilizers farmers apply to their fields—it is the excess fertilizer, not absorbed by plants, that washes into streams or percolates into groundwater. Through some complex of social and economic arrangements, farmers might be persuaded to use less fertilizer and more humus. By improving the texture of soils, as well as providing slowly released nutrients, humus can reduce the need for commercial fertilizer to keep up crop yields. The U.S. produces enormous quantities of organic wastes that could be converted to humus. Such a remedy for fertilizer pollution, of course, might seem highly undesirable to the fertilizer industry, already burdened with excess capacity.

DISPENSING WITH BACTERIA

Even if phosphorus pollution from fertilizers and detergents were entirely eliminated—an unlikely prospect—phosphates from domestic and industrial wastes would still impose a heavy load upon rivers and lakes. As population and industry grow, higher and higher percentages of the phosphorus will have to be removed from effluents to keep the algae problem from getting worse. The conventional technology being pushed by the federal water-pollution war cannot cope with phosphorus, or with many other pollutants. But there are advanced technologies that can. Advanced water treatment, sometimes called "tertiary," is generally aimed at removal of all, or almost all, of the contaminants.

One promising idea under investigation is to dispense with the not always reliable bacteria that consume sewage in secondary treatment. Toxic industrial wastes have on occasion thrown municipal treatment plants out of kilter for weeks by killing the bacteria. "We've found that we can accomplish the same kind of treatment with a purely physical-chemical process," says a scientist at the Robert A. Taft Water Research Center in Cincinnati.

In this new approach, the raw sewage is clarified with chemicals to remove most suspended organic material, including much of the phosphate. Then comes carbon adsorption. The effluent passes through filter beds of granular activated carbon, similar to that used in charcoal filters for cigarettes. Between clarification and adsorption, 90 percent or more of the phosphate is removed. The carbon can be regenerated in furnaces and reused. Captured organic matter is burned. Carbon adsorption has the great additional advantage of removing from the water organic industrial chemicals that pass unhindered through biological secondary treatment. The chemicals adhere to the carbon as they swirl through its complex structure with millions of pathways and byways.

A PRODUCT RATHER THAN AN EFFLUENT

Other treatment techniques are under study that make water even cleaner, and might possibly be used to turn sewage into potable water. One of these is reverse osmosis, originally developed for demineralization of brackish water. When liquids with different concentrations of, say, mineral salts are separated by a semipermeable membrane, water molecules pass by osmosis, a natural equalizing tendency, from the less concentrated to the more concentrated side to create an equilibrium. In reverse osmosis, strong pressure is exerted on the side with the greater concentration. The pressure reverses the natural flow, forcing molecules of pure water through the membrane, out of the high-salt or high-particle concentration. Reverse osmosis removes ammonia nitrogen, as well as phosphates, most nitrate, and other substances dissolved in water. Unfortunately, the process is not yet applicable to sewage treatment on a large scale because the membranes become fouled with sewage solids. Engineers are hard at work trying to design better membranes.

New techniques are gradually transforming sewage treatment, technically backward and sometimes poorly controlled, into something akin to a modern chemical process. "We are talking about a wedding of sanitary and chemical engineering," says David G. Stephan, who directs research and development at the Federal Water Pollution Control Administration, "using the techniques of the chemical process industry to turn out a product—reusable water—rather than an effluent to throw away." Adds James McDermott of the Public Health Service: "We're going to get to the point where, on the one hand, it's going to cost us an awful lot of money to treat wastes and dump them into the stream. And an awful lot of money to take those wastes when they are going down the stream and make drinking water out of them. We are eventually going to create treatment plants where we take sewage and, instead of dumping it back into the stream, treat it with a view of recycling it immediately—direct reuse. That is the only way we're going to satisfy our water needs, and second, it's going to be cheaper."

Windhoek, the capital of arid South West Africa, last year gained the distinction of becoming the first city in the world to recycle its waste water directly into drinking water. Waste water is taken out of sewers, processed conventionally, oxidized in ponds for about a month, then run through filters and activated-carbon columns, chlorinated, and put back into the water mains. Windhoek's distinction may prove to be dubious, because the full effects of recycled water on health are unknown. There is a potential hazard of viruses (hepatitis, polio, etc.) being concentrated in recycling. For this reason many health experts feel that renovated sewage should not be accepted as drinking water in the U.S. until its safety can be more reliably demonstrated.

Costs naturally go up as treatment gets more complex. While primary-secondary treatment costs about 12 cents a thousand gallons of waste water, the advanced techniques in use at Lake Tahoe, for instance, bring the cost up to 30 cents. About 7½ cents of the increase is for phosphorus removal. Reverse osmosis at this stage would raise the cost to at least 35 cents a thousand gallons, higher than the average cost of drinking water to metered households in the U.S. Whatever new techniques are accepted, rising costs of pollution control will be a fact of life.

A PERFECT MARRIAGE FOR SLUDGE

Ironically, these new treatment techniques, such as removal of phosphorus with chemicals, will intensify one of the most pressing operational problems in waste-water treatment—sludge disposal. Sludge, the solid matter removed from domestic or industrial waste water, is a nuisance, highly contaminated unless it's disinfected. The handling and disposal of sludge can eat up to one-half of a treatment plant's operating budget. Some communities incinerate their sludge, contributing to air pollution. "Now in cleaning the water further we are adding chemicals to take out phosphorus and more solids," says Francis M. Middleton, director of the Taft Center. "While we end up with cleaner water, we also end up with even greater quantities of sludge."

Chicago's struggle with its sludge illustrates some of the difficulties and perhaps an effective way of coping with them. With 1,000 tons of sludge a day to dispose of, the metropolitan sanitary district has been stuffing about half of it into deep holes near treatment plants, at a cost of about $60 a ton. The other half is dried and shipped to Florida and elsewhere where it is sold to citrus growers and companies producing fertilizers for $12 a ton—a nonprofit operation. Vinton W. Bacon, general superintendent of the sanitary district, says this state of affairs can't continue. "We're running out of land. Not only that, but the land we're using for disposal is valuable. And even it will be filled within two years."

Bacon is convinced he has an answer that will not only cut costs but also solve disposal problems indefinitely while helping to make marginal lands bloom. Bacon's scheme, tested in pilot projects in Chicago and elsewhere, is to pump liquid sludge through a pipeline to strip mines and marginal farmland about sixty miles southwest of Chicago. "We put the sludge water through tanks where it's digested," Bacon says. "Then it can be used directly without any odor or health dangers. It's the perfect marriage. That land needs our sludge as much as we need the land. Most astounding, even acquiring the required land at current market prices, taking in the cost of a twenty-four-inch, sixty-mile-long pipeline, the pumps, reservoirs, irrigation equipment, and manpower, the cost would still come to only $20 a ton. We could build a pipeline 200 miles long and still not run higher costs than with our present system."

An aspect of water pollution that seems harder to cope with is the overflow of combined sewers during storms. A combined system that unites storm and sanitary sewers into a single network usually has interceptor sewers, with direct outlets to a stream, to protect the treatment plant from flooding during heavy rains. But in diverting excess water from treatment plants, interceptor sewers dump raw sewage into the waterways. Obviously, this partly defeats the purpose of having treatment plants.

So bad are the consequences of sewer overflow that some specialists would prefer to see part of the federal money that is being channeled into secondary treatment go into correction of the combined-sewer problem instead. But more than 1,300 U.S. communities have combined sewers, and the cost of separating the systems would be huge. The American Public Works Association estimated the cost of total separation at $48 *billion.* The job could be done in an alternative fashion for a still shocking $15 billion, by building holding tanks for the overflow storm water. Still another possibility would be to build separate systems for sewage and to use existing sewers for storm water. The federal war on water pollution discourages construction of combined sewers but strangely includes no money (except for $28 million already awarded for research and development) to remedy the problem of existing combined-sewer systems.

SLICING UP RIVERS

The General Accounting Office recently surveyed federal activities in water-pollution control and found some glaring deficiencies. The G.A.O. prepared its report for Congress and therefore failed to point out that in some of the deficiencies the real culprit was Congress itself. Still largely rural-oriented, Congress originally limited federal grants for construction of waste-treatment facilities to $250,000 per municipality. The dollar ceiling was eventually raised, but was not removed until fiscal 1968. In the preceding twelve years about half of the waste-treatment facilities were built in hamlets with populations of less than 2,500, and 92 percent in towns with populations under 50,000.

In drafting the legislation that provides for new water-quality standards, Congress again showed limited vision, leaving it up to the states to decide many important questions. Each state is free to make its own decisions on pollution-control goals in terms of determining the uses to which a particular stream or lake will be put. Each state is to decide on the stream characteristics that would allow such uses—dissolved oxygen, temperature, etc. Finally, each state is to set up a schedule for corrective measures that would ensure the stream quality decided upon, and prepare plans for legal enforcement of the standards.

It would have been logical to set standards for entire river basins since rivers don't always stay within state boundaries. What's more, there were already several regional river-basin compacts in existence that could have taken on the job. But with the single exception of the Delaware River Basin Commission, of which the federal government is a member, the government bypassed the regional bodies and insisted that each state set its own standards. Predictably, the result has been confusion. The states submitted standards by June 30,1967, but Interior has given full approval to only twenty-five states and territories. It has now become the prickly task of the Secretary of the Interior to reconcile the conflicting sets of standards that states have established for portions of the same rivers.

Some states facing each other across a river have set different standards for water characteristics, as if dividing the river flow in the middle with a bureaucratic fence. Kentucky and Indiana, across the Ohio from each other, submitted two different temperature standards for that river: Kentucky came up with a maximum of 93° Fahrenheit, while Indiana wants 90°. Similarly, Ohio set its limit at 93°, while West Virginia, across the same river, chose 86°. Up the river, Pennsylvania, too, decided on 86°. One reason for such differences about river temperature is that biologists don't always agree among themselves about safe temperatures for aquatic life. At one recent meeting in Cincinnati, where federal and state officials were attempting to reconcile the different figures for the Ohio, the disagreement among biologists was so great that one exasperated engineer suggested, "Maybe we should start putting ice cubes at different points in the river."

A FAILURE OF IMAGINATION

The biggest deficiency in the federal approach is its lack of imagination. Congress chose the subsidy route as being the easiest, but the task could have been undertaken much more thoughtfully. A regional or river-valley approach would have required more careful working out than a program of state-by-state standards and subsidies, but it would have made more sense economically, and would have assured continuing management of water quality.

A promising river-valley program is evolving along the Great Miami River in Ohio. The Miami Conservancy District, a regional flood-control agency, began two years ago to explore the concept of river management. The Great Miami runs through a heavily industrialized valley. There are, for instance, eighteen paper mills in the valley. Dayton, the principal city on the river, houses four divisions of General Motors and is the home of National Cash Register. To finance a three-year exploratory program, the Miami Conservancy District has imposed temporary charges, based on volume of effluent, on sixty plants, businesses, and municipalities along the river. These charges amount to a total of $350,000 a year, ranging from $500 that might be paid by a motel to $23,000 being paid by a single power-generating station.

With this money, plus a $500,000 grant for the Federal Water Pollution Control Administration, the district has been looking into river-wide measures that will be needed to control pollution even *after* every municipality along the river has a secondary treatment plant. (Dayton already has one.) The district's staff of sanitary engineers, ecologists, and systems analysts has come up with suggested measures to augment the low flow of the river as an additional method of pollution control. The Great Miami's mean annual flow at Dayton is 2,500 cubic feet a second, but every ten years or so it falls to a mere 170 cubic feet a second. To assure a more even flow, the Miami District will build either reservoirs or facilities to pump ground water, at a cost of several million dollars. The cost will be shared by river users. District engineers are also exploring in-stream aeration, or artificial injection of air into the river to provide additional dissolved oxygen. The state has set an ambitious goal for the Great Miami—to make the river usable "for all purposes, at all places, all the time."

To meet this goal, the district will introduce waste-discharge fees, which will probably be based on the amount of oxygen-demanding wastes or hot water discharged. Will these amount to a charge for polluting the river? "No," says Max L. Mitchell, the district's chief engineer. "Charges will be high enough to make industry reduce water use."

Federal money would do a lot more good if it were divided up along the river-basin lines instead of municipality by municipality or state by state, with little regard for differences in pollution at different points in a basin. To distribute federal funds more effectively, Congress would have to overcome its parochial orientation. Also, Congress should be channeling more funds into new waste-treatment technologies and ways of putting them to use. Unless pollution abatement is undertaken in an imaginative and systematic manner, the "war" against dirty rivers may be a long, losing campaign.

Solid Wastes

Solid wastes etch a trail of visible blight that leaves few corners of the country unspotted. Across the Nation the same scenes repeat—refuse in the streets, litter on beaches and along roadsides, abandoned autos on isolated curbsides and in weeded vacant lots, rusty refrigerators and stoves in backyards, thousands of dumps scarring the landscape. And the less visible aspects of the problem—solid wastes in the ocean, contamination of ground water, and wasted resources—are just as critical. America's well-known penchant for convenience has come face-to-face with major environmental problems.

Proper management of solid wastes is a key to upgrading environmental quality. Stricter enforcement of air quality standards has focused attention on burning dumps and inefficient incinerators, many of them operated by municipal governments. Water quality research is beginning to probe the effects of dumps and landfills on the purity of ground water.

Public appreciation of the magnitude of the economic and social costs of solid waste is building and a concept of solid waste management is evolving. It assumes that man can devise a social-technological system that will wisely control the quantity and characteristics of wastes, efficiently collect those that must be removed, creatively recycle those that can be reused, and properly dispose of those that have no further use.

The growing technology and affluence of American society have laid a heavy burden on solid waste facilities. Refuse collected in urban areas of the Nation has increased from 2.75 pounds per person per day in 1920 to 5 pounds in 1970. It is expected to reach 8 pounds by 1980. This spiraling volume of solid waste has a changing character. The trend toward packaged goods in disposable containers has put more paper, plastics, glass, and metals instead of organic matter into the refuse. And technology of solid waste collection and disposal has not kept pace with this change.

There has been little attempt to tie the production of consumer goods together with the disposability of those parts that end as waste. Disposal costs are not included in the price paid by the consumer; rather they are borne by

Excerpt from *Environmental Quality,* The First Annual Report of the Council on Environmental Quality, Transmitted to the Congress, August 1970.

society in general. With few exceptions manufacturers do not accept responsibility for the costs of getting rid of products that have been sold and served their purpose.

Solid waste collection in most municipalities is inadequate and antiquated, partly because over the years it has endured more than its share of public neglect. Refuse collection jobs are low status and low paying, and injury statistics show that only logging is a more hazardous occupation. Sanitation workers have been striking with increasing frequency, and heaps of reeking wastes have been left for days on curbsides in our largest cities. This has dramatized the human factors in the business of refuse collection. It has pointed up the close correlation between the working conditions of trash collectors and the public health menace of inadequate collection and disposal.

Disposal facilities are equally inadequate and antiquated. The Bureau of Solid Waste Management of the Department of Health, Education, and Welfare estimates that 94 percent of existing land disposal operations and 75 percent of incinerator facilities are substandard.

WHAT MAKES SOLID WASTES

The total solid wastes produced in the United States in 1969 reached 4.3 billion tons as shown in the following table:

	Million tons
Residential, Commercial and Institutional wastes	250
Collected	(190)
Uncollected	(60)
Industrial wastes	110
Mineral wastes	1,700
Agricultural wastes	2,280
Total	4,340

Sources : Bureau of Solid Waste Management, Department of Health, Education, and Welfare ; Division of Solid Wastes, Bureau of Mines, Department of the Interior.

Most of it originated from agriculture and livestock. Other large amounts arose from mining and industrial processes. A little under 6 percent, or 250 million tons, was classified as residential, commercial, and institutional solid wastes. And only three-fourths of this was collected.

Although wastes from homes, businesses, and institutions make up a small part of the total load of solid waste produced, they are the most offensive and the most dangerous to health when they accumulate near where people live. Agricultural and mineral wastes, although much greater in volume, are generally spread more widely over the land. They are more isolated from population concentrations and may not require special collection and disposal. Nevertheless, as more is learned about the effects of agricultural and mineral wastes on the quality of air, water, and esthetics, steps to curb their production and facilitate disposal seem likely.

The largest single source of solid wastes in this country is agriculture. It accounts for over half the total. The more than 2 billion tons of *agricultural wastes* produced each year includes animal and slaughterhouse wastes, useless residues from crop harvesting, vineyard and orchard prunings, and greenhouse wastes.

Herds of cattle and other animals, once left to graze over large open meadows, are now often confined to feedlots where they fatten more rapidly for market. On these feedlots, they generate enormous and concentrated quantities of manure that cannot readily and safely be assimilated by the soil. Manure permeates the earth and invades waterbodies, contributing to fish kills, eutrophied lakes, off-flavored drinking waters, and contaminated aquifers. Feedlots intensify odors, dusts, and the wholesale production of flies and other noxious insects. Animal waste disposal is a growing problem because the demand for animal manure as a soil conditioner is declining. Easier handling, among other advantages, favors chemical fertilizers.

About 110 million tons of *industrial solid wastes* (excluding mineral solid wastes) are generated every year. More than 15 million tons of it are scrap metal, and 30 million tons are paper and paper product wastes; a miscellaneous bag of slags, waste plastics, bales of rags, and drums of assorted products discarded for various reasons make up the rest. The electric utility industry produced over 30 million tons of fly ash in 1969 from burning bituminous coal and lignite. By 1980, the figure could rise to 40 million tons. Currently, only about 20 percent of ash material finds any use.

In the past year, 1,700 million tons of *mineral solid wastes,* comprising 39 percent of total solid wastes, were generated in the United States—most of it from the mineral and fossil fuel mining, milling, and processing industries. Slag heaps, culm piles, and mill tailings accumulate near extraction or processing operations. Eighty mineral industries generate solid waste, but only eight of them are responsible for 80 percent of the total. Copper contributes the largest waste tonnage, followed by iron and steel, bituminous coal, phosphate rock, lead, zinc, alumina, and anthracite. By 1980, the Nation's mineral industries will be generating at least 2 billion tons of waste every year.

In 1969, Americans threw away more than 250 million tons of *residential, commercial, and institutional solid wastes.* Approximately 190 million tons were collected by public agencies and private refuse firms. The remainder was abandoned, dumped, disposed of at the point of origin, or hauled away by the producer to a disposal site. About $3.5 billion was spent last year handling the 190 million tons of collected solid wastes—an average of $18 per ton. Collection accounts for 80 percent of the cost ($14 per ton), disposal for the rest. A considerably higher rate of spending would be needed to upgrade existing systems to acceptable levels of operation.

The solid waste collected annually includes 30 million tons of paper and paper products; 4 million tons of plastics; 100 million tires; 30 billion bottles; 60 billion cans; millions of tons of demolition debris, grass and tree trimmings, food wastes, and sewage sludge; and millions of discarded automobiles and major appliances.

COLLECTION AND DISPOSAL

Residential, commercial, institutional, and industrial solid wastes are the clearest threats to health and to the environment. So they are the chief target of the waste disposal strategy. Most such waste comes from the urban areas and requires quick removal. It is increasing at a rate of about 4 percent a year.

Three facets of the production and discard of these growing mountains of solid waste materials need examination : solid waste handling, natural resource depletion, and litter and abandonment. Collection and disposal costs continue to spiral. This is partly because of wage hikes—to bring the pay of sanitation workers more into line with other occupations. But even more, it is to pay for new collection equipment and landfill and dumping sites and, in some communities, to amortize incineration equipment. Researchers are beginning to examine what is entering the solid waste stream. Ultimately they hope to reduce unnecessary discard or even to restrict the manufacture of some items.

Natural resource management requires that minerals in shortest supply be identified and efforts made to cut the quantity discarded and to recycle whatever is collected. Some key minerals are already recycled to a considerable extent. More lead is pulled from scrap than from mined ores, and nearly half of the copper used today comes from scrap. However, for many natural resources, substantial Federal income tax incentives and other laws and policies encourage use of the virgin material instead and undercut the competitive position of recycled materials.

The litter problem—tires, bottles, cans, plastics, and paper thrown away randomly instead of into waste containers—adds daily to collection costs and blight. Many of the nation's roads, beaches, rivers, parks, and other public areas are cluttered with the refuse of thoughtless citizens. Litter collection costs average $88 per ton, more than four times as much as collecting residential refuse.

Collection Methods

Refuse collection methods in most of the United States do not differ substantially from what they were when workers picked up the trash in horse-drawn wagons before the turn of the century. This lack of technological advance is particularly burdensome because up to 80 percent of the funds spent on solid waste management goes into collecting the waste and hauling it to a processing plant or a dump.

The one significant advance has been the compactor truck. These closed-body vehicles now make up a large part of the 150,000 refuse collection trucks in the United States. With hydraulic presses, they compress waste, usually at a 3-to-1 ratio, thus saving vehicle space and cutting the number of trips necessary to cover collection routes. However, the compactor has disadvantages. Because refuse of different types is mixed and crushed, recyclables are lost or contaminated by unusable waste. It is also hazardous to operators.

Efforts are underway to modernize trash collection. Under one Federal grant, researchers at The Johns Hopkins University are studying the practicability of transfer points in waste collection systems serving large cities. Under another, the University of Pennsylvania is studying the possibility of pipelines for collecting and removing domestic solid wastes. The pipeline method may be technologically feasible and economically attractive. But these are just beginnings. More research is mandatory.

Disposal Techniques

The final disposal point for an estimated 77 percent of all collected solid wastes is 14,000 open dumps in the country. Thirteen percent is deposited into properly operated sanitary landfills, where wastes are adequately covered each day with earth of the proper type. Nearly all of the remaining 10 percent is burned. Incinerators are used primarily in large cities, where the volume of refuse and the high cost of land make incineration an attractive disposal method. Small quantities of solid wastes are turned into nutrient-rich soil conditioners by composting operations. And a small but troublesome percentage is dumped at sea.

Land disposal of solid wastes can range from the most offensive fly-and rat-infested open dump to technically advanced practices that end in the creation of parklands, golf courses, outdoor theaters, and other public facilities. Disposal sites in or near urban areas can be reclaimed for use as attractive open space if proper sanitary landfill practices are employed.

Imaginative thinking in land disposal practices is not widespread. Collected refuse is dumped in whatever area is available, with little or no provision for soil cover. Often city fathers blame spontaneous combustion for fires at these dumps. But in at least some cases, local sanitation officials set fire to wastes to reduce their volume because dumps are overloaded. Burning at open dumps remains a major cause of air pollution in some cities. Improper landfill techniques can spawn large quantities of methane gas and breed armies of rats, flies, and other pests. Disposal sites often mar wetlands and scenic areas. Some

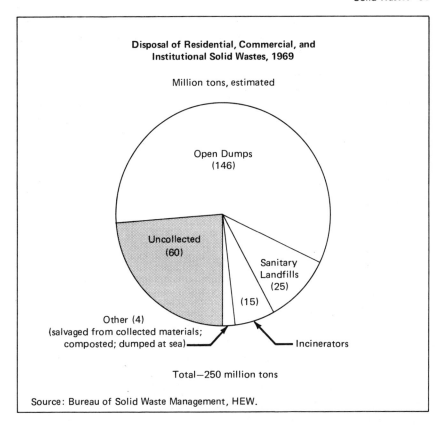

Disposal of Residential, Commercial, and Institutional Solid Wastes, 1969

Million tons, estimated

Open Dumps
(146)

Uncollected
(60)

Sanitary
Landfills
(25)

(15)

Other (4)
(salvaged from collected materials;
composted; dumped at sea)

Incinerators

Total—250 million tons

Source: Bureau of Solid Waste Management, HEW.

are uneconomical because of their distance from the city. In California, filling canyons and other natural areas has been censored by conservation groups.

Improved equipment for landfilling is being developed. For example, with a grant from the Bureau of Solid Waste Management, King County (Seattle), Wash., is constructing a machine called the "Mole," which will compact refuse at high pressure and dispose of it below ground level. Under another grant, a landfill operation near Virginia Beach, Va., will be turned into a huge manmade hill for an amphitheater. A similar site near Chicago will be developed for tobogganing and skiing.

The city of Madison, Wis., has a grant to build and operate a hammer reduction mill to test the economic feasibility of salvaging paper and metals. Preliminary investigations of salvage possibilities are inconclusive, but disposal aspects of the mill look promising. It may be possible, for example, that milled refuse may safely be deposited in a landfill without earth cover.

Strip mining for coal has scarred some landscapes in the United States and left them denuded of vegetation and open to erosion. Several years ago rail haul of solid wastes was proposed as a solution to two environmental problems—unsightly abandoned strip mines and the shortage of disposal sites near large eastern cities. The plan involved using railroad dump cars which usually return from cities to mining sites empty. Many factors, including outlying community resistance to taking in other people's refuse have limited that idea. But disposal costs in large cities have shot up so sharply that the concept is being reconsidered. A Federal grant has been awarded to the American Public Works Association to investigate hauling refuse by rail from large urban areas to remote, mined areas for landfilling.

Nearly 10 percent of domestic solid wastes is processed through *incineration;* 300 municipal incinerators account for about half the tonnage burned; the rest is consumed in thousands of small, privately owned trash burners. After incineration, about 25 percent of the waste by weight remains—as ashes, glass, metals, and unburned combustibles. These then must be removed and recycled, or disposed of in some way.

Since municipal incineration is often cited as a polluter of air, research is underway to improve incinerator technology. A German process involves a mechanically stoked rotary drum incinerator designed for small communities. West Virginia University is studying a fluidized-bed incinerator fueled by mixtures of domestic and industrial solid wastes.

One of the most promising engineering concepts in solid waste management is the CPU–400, now under development by the Combustion Power Co. of Palo Alto, Calif. The CPU–400 is a fluidized-bed incinerator, which burns solid waste at high pressure, which produces hot gases, which power a turbine, which in turn drives an electric generator. Municipal solid wastes constitute a better fuel than might have been expected. They have a heating value of 5,000 British thermal units per pound—about one-third that of a good grade of coal. Municipal wastes are also low in sulfur, a major air pollution source. As designed, the CPU–400 should produce approximately 15,000 kilowatts of electric power daily, while burning 400 tons of municipal refuse. The generator unit should supply 10 percent of the electric power requirements of the community providing the refuse. Up to three-fourths of the heat in the gas turbine cycle is available for auxiliary functions such as steam production, sewage sludge drying, or perhaps saline water conversion. The CPU–400 concept also envisions using the vacuum produced by the gas turbine to draw refuse to the incinerator from collection points in the city—through pipes buried in the streets.

The Bureau of Mines of the Department of the Interior is applying the process of carbonization (destructive distillation) to the disposal of industrial wastes and urban refuse. This process involves the thermal conversion of materials into usable forms of solid, liquid, and gaseous products.

An insignificant amount of collected solid wastes in the United States is *composted.* Metals, glass, and similar inorganics are sorted from mixed refuse, and the remainder is converted to a peat-like organic fertilizer and soil conditioner. This process is widely used in Europe. Madrid composts 200 tons daily and Moscow is opening a new 600-ton-per-day facility. Composting has never been popular in the United States for several reasons. Compared to many Western European nations, land available for disposal sites in the United States is inexpensive. The compost product has not always been of uniform quality here; nor has it competed with commercial soil conditioners. Also, the composition of refuse in the United States makes it more difficult to compost, since its organic content is low. Finally, composting was first sold to American cities as a profitmaking venture. When it did not pay off, many cities considered the enterprise a failure. The Bureau of Solid Waste Management, jointly with the Tennessee Valley Authority, is operating an experimental composting plant in Johnson City, Tenn. But the results have not been encouraging. In recent years almost all composting plants in this country have shut down.

Some coastal cities and industries are turning to *ocean disposal* to get rid of solid waste. Lack of suitable land disposal sites and stricter air pollution standards for incinerators make ocean dumping look attractive. In his April 15 Message on Waste Disposal, the President directed the Council on Environmental Quality to report to him by September 1, 1970, on environmental problems associated with ocean dumping.

RECYCLING AND REUSE

In his February 10 Message on the Environment, the President announced the Federal Government's goal to reduce solid waste volume and encourage reuse and recycling. Recycling waste materials into the economy has not been widely applied in the United States. Economic considerations and the abundance of virgin resources have forestalled the development of recycling technology and markets. Primary materials producers, often with the help of tax concessions, have developed remarkable efficient technologies for removing metals and other substances from their virgin state. But meanwhile, techniques for separating and recovering waste materials remain primitive and expensive.

There are many aspects to recycling. The characteristics and the volume of the products which enter the market and eventually end up as solid wastes are one. Identification of characteristics and items most troublesome to solid waste management is another. And decisions on how to control their presence in refuse are still another. Some items can be returned by consumers for reuse. Others may be sorted by householders for separate collection. Or the most economical solution may be to salvage from mixed collection wastes.

Sorting Mixed Refuse

Much more work is needed to develop an effective way to salvage the valuable elements of collected mixed refuse. It is difficult and costly. And the instability of salvage markets has only added to the problem. The Stanford Research Institute in Menlo Park, Calif., has constructed a pilot scale unit in which a vertical stream of air separates mixed waste materials. After technical difficulties are overcome, this air classification process may prove an economic alternative to hand separation.

At College Park, Md., the Bureau of Mines has constructed an advanced reclamation system with mechanical separators which sort metals and glass from incinerator residues. Recent technological advances there have produced a highly sophisticated process which sorts glass by color and isolates several exotic metals. It adds $3 per ton to normal collection and disposal costs, not considering any income from the sale of salvaged materials. The Bureau is now developing data for the design of commercial plants based on this process.

Auto Disposal

A number of specific components in solid wastes present particular problems and require special mention. Abandoned autos are one of the most conspicuous solid waste disposal problems. On the average, 9 million autos are retired from service every year. Although statistics on the annual number of abandoned vehicles are subject to dispute, it is thought that approximately 15 percent are abandoned on city streets, in back alleys, along rural roads, and in vacant lots throughout the Nation. Most autos are abandoned because they are no longer serviceable and have little or no parts value to auto wreckers. The total number of abandoned cars in the country is even harder to ascertain, but has been estimated between 2.5 and 4.5 million.

The 85 percent of autos that are properly turned in by their owners enter a complex recycling system, usually beginning with the auto wrecker, whose chief business is selling the parts that can be removed. Some wreckers claim to obtain 97 percent of their sales revenues from parts. The high value of junk cars for parts and their often negligible value for scrap means that wreckers have little incentive to move their inventories to scrap processors. Except when there is demand for scrap, the junk cars just pile up.

Auto wreckers eventually, however, have to move the hulks to scrap processors. Most processors, using powerful hydraulic presses, reduce the cars to small bales containing high percentages of nonferrous materials—copper, upholstery, chrome, plastic, and glass. The bales are then sold to steel mills, which turn them into products which do not require high quality steel, or pass them on to mills which have sufficient capacity to dilute their contaminants. A growing number of processors produce a higher priced scrap through mechanical shredding and electromagnetic separation. Costs for shredding equipment, however, have limited the widespread use of this process, particularly by small scrap processors.

Steel mills and foundries are major users of ferrous scrap. In 1969, 50 percent of the material used for the production of all steel products was scrap. Six percent of that scrap was from junk autos. But changes in steel production techniques make it difficult to predict future scrap needs. Basic oxygen furnaces and electrical induction furnaces are partially replacing the open hearth furnace. The first requires less scrap, but the second uses more. It is even more difficult to predict export scrap demand and the effects of new fabricating and casting processes on the scrap market.

In his February 10 Message on the Environment, the President asked the Council on Environmental Quality to take the lead in recommending a bounty payment or some other system to promote the prompt scrapping of all junk automobiles. The Council has reviewed the range of alternatives leading to a Federal or State bounty system and concluded that under present conditions it is not practicable.

Most of the systems considered by the Council would be funded by a tax on the sale of all automobiles sold in the future or the collection of a fee from all present owners and future buyers. The bounty payment would be made to the scrap processor, the auto wrecker, or the owner of the car being junked. All of these proposals would put an unfair burden on the owners of the 85 percent of autos that are properly turned over to auto wreckers, in order to take care of the remainder which are not. Furthermore, the Council is not persuaded that the demand for auto scrap would be improved by such a system, nor that it would in fact influence the economics affecting abandonment. The resulting fund of payments would divert billions of dollars from other investments in the private economy. Administration and enforcement of the system would require excessive increases in government personnel and expenditures. The Council also determined that firm penalties against abandonment and improvement of State title and transfer laws alone, particularly for cars of low value, might substantially reduce abandonment and put abandoned vehicles more promptly into the scrapping cycle. Such laws should be strengthened.

Any attempt to solve the problem of abandoned cars, however, must consider the problems of fluctuating scrap demand, steel production technology, transportation rates for scrap, export scrap markets, availability of shredding equipment, and characteristics of the auto parts market. Otherwise, assuming abandonment could be reversed, hulks would only continue to pile up in junk yards. The Council will continue its study of these broader problems, looking toward a solution that will involve the entire auto scrapping system.

Other Items

In 1969, 43.8 billion *beverage containers* for beer and soft drinks were made in the United States. If the trend to throw-away containers continues, by 1980,

100 billion of these bottles and cans will be produced and discarded every year. Beverage containers already comprise 3.9 percent of all collected refuse, and the number is growing at a rate of nearly 7.5 percent per year—compared to 4 percent for all refuse. Bottles and cans constitute a major part of what is left in incinerators after burning. They must be hauled to land disposal sites. Each year an estimated 1 to 2 billion glass and metal beverage containers end up as litter on highways, beaches, parks, and other public areas. Severe penalties for littering have not worked in the face of the rising sales of the throw-away bottle and can, and strict enforcement of these laws has been difficult.

Paper constitutes almost 60 percent of roadside litter and is difficult to collect. Last year, 58.3 million tons of paper were consumed in the United States. Nineteen percent of this was recycled. Fifteen percent was temporarily retained or lost its identity in manufacturing processes. The remaining two-thirds—or 40 million tons—was discarded as residential, commercial, institutional, and industrial solid wastes. Typically, paper comprising 40 to 50 percent of mixed refuse is disposed of at an annual cost of over $900 million. Paper production is a multiple polluter. It crops up as a factor in timber wastes, in air and water pollution, and in the removal of organic materials from soils in managed forests. Much of the discarded paper consists of technically reusable fiber. Although the United States recycles only 19 percent of its paper, Japan reclaims and reprocesses nearly half of the paper its people use.

Plastics comprise an increasingly worrisome element in solid wastes. They are virtually indestructible, do not degrade naturally, and resist the compression plates of compactor trucks. In incinerators most plastics tend to melt rather than burn and to foul the grates. One range of plastics, polyvinyl chloride (PVC), is a new arrival in the packaging market. When burned, it produces hydrochloric acid. Although not yet widely used in the United States, in Germany it has already been blamed for increased air pollution, damage to incinerator stacks, and—in rare cases—destruction of nearby flora.

Another potential problem arises from disposing of *pesticides.* As stronger legislation and regulation of these agents take effect, the proper disposal of undesirable or condemned commodities becomes important. Even the containers used to market pesticides may retain considerable toxicity after discard. Although there have as yet been no serious cases, concentration of these agents in sanitary landfills and open dumps could contaminate ground water and imperil public health.

Rubber tires are just as difficult to get rid of. Burning them pollutes the air. In sanitary landfills, they defy compaction and tend to gravitate to the surface. Changing technology has lessened the use of old rubber in the manufacture of new rubber products; thus most old tires are not recycled.

The Fish and Wildlife Service and the Bureau of Solid Waste Management are investigating the use of old tires as reefs and fish havens along the Atlantic coast of the United States. The ocean bottom is sandy and relatively flat for great distances. And artificial reefs constructed of tires may promote an increase in desirable species since many game fish require relief features such as reefs for protection and spawning grounds. If this concept proves practical, very large numbers of old tires could be turned into an important ecological side benefit.

IV. UNDERSTANDING NOISE

AND

RADIATION POLLUTION

Sound Pollution — Another Urban Problem

Peter A. Breysse

In a recent article entitled "Noise and Urban Man," Robert Alex Baron states:

> Noise abatement and the need for it are virtually neglected issues in American life today. Unless the medical and public health professions become deeply involved in these problems, it is likely that apathy and inertia will defer any effective action for another decade or even longer. But we, the public, cannot wait that long. Air pollution kills us slowly but silently; noise makes each day a torment.[1]

Noise, defined as "unwanted sound," surrounds today's urban dweller in an excessive and gradually increasing diet of decibels. While it is generally accepted that noise is unwanted sound, there is no universally agreed-upon definition for sound pollution. Sound pollution may be defined as the presence in the environment of noise resulting from human activities, which is of sufficient quantity and quality to adversely affect man's well-being, either physiologically or psychologically and/or interfere with man's full use and enjoyment of his property.

To fully appreciate the complexity of the sound pollution problem, we may need to review briefly this phenomenon called sound. Sound consists of a series of vibrations in an elastic medium. A vibrating body, such as a guitar string, produces compression waves. As these waves emanate from the vibrating body, molecules of the transmitting medium—air, for example—are alternately compressed and expanded (Figure 1). Thus, sound is transmitted through compressible matter. Sound waves generally travel faster in dense materials. The velocity of sound in air is 1,130 feet per second (ft/sec); in water, 4,500 ft/sec; and in steel, 15,000 ft/sec.

When sound is transmitted through the atmosphere, the vibrations may impinge upon the human ear which, if functioning properly, transmits the physical energy to the auditory nerves. The normal ear distinguishes between

Reprinted by permission from *The Science Teacher*, April 1970, pp. 25-34.
(Adapted from a talk given at the 1969 NSTA regional conference in Seattle.)
[1]Baron, Robert Alex. "Noise and Urban Man," *American Journal of Public Health* 58 : 2060-2066; November 1968.

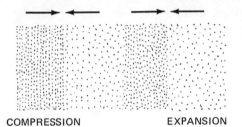

Figure 1. Alternate compression and expansion of molecules of the transmitting medium creates sound waves.

COMPRESSION   EXPANSION

sounds by detecting the different tones of which each sound is composed. The audible tones (Figure 2) range from approximately 16 Hertz (HZ) to 16,000 HZ (HZ = cycles per second). The principal speech range extends from approximately 300 to 3,500 HZ. At the lower and upper ends of the spectrum, higher energies are necessary to discern these sounds. Below 16 HZ we are in the region of vibrations, and above 20,000 HZ in the ultrasonic region. The threshold of discomfort begins at 120 decibels (db) and the threshold of pain at 130 db.

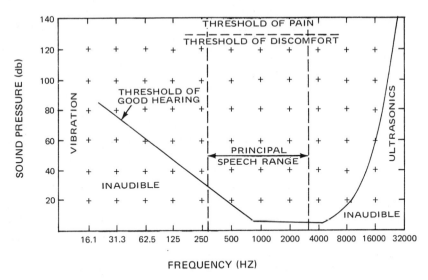

Figure 2. The auditory field of humans ranges from approximately 16 to 16,000 cycles per second.

The characteristic sounds of the urban environment consist of pure tones (sound of single frequency) and random sounds (those with no consistent tone, such as a waterfall). This combination of pure tones and random sounds forms what are called complex sounds.

The human ear is an amazing instrument. It can recognize and classify approximately 340,000 separate tones, and it can hear without damage a sound pressure 10 million times greater than the sound pressure of the softest intelligible sound. Because of this wide range of responses, a system of logarithms is utilized to measure sound intensity. Originally, sound intensity was defined in terms of sound power. Because sound power cannot be measured directly and sound pressure can, power was converted to pressure such that:

$$\text{Sound Pressure Level (db)} = 20 \log_{10} \frac{\text{Measured Pressure}}{\text{Reference Pressure}}$$

$$\text{(SPL)}$$

Reference Pressure
$$= \ 0.0002 \ (\text{dynes}/\text{cm}^2)$$

Source	SPL (db)
Jet plane (100 ft)	140
Riveter	120
Rock and roll music	120
Cub Scout meeting (at times)	110
Subway train (inside)	95-110
Automobile (inside— window open)	95-110
City traffic	90-110
Normal conversation	60-70
Quiet office	40-60
Whisper	40-60
Threshold of hearing	0[a]

[a]This differs for individuals.

Since SPL is based on a logarithmic relationship, intensities of multiple sources cannot be added arithmetically. The additive effect of two SPLs of the same magnitude would theoretically increase the SPL 6 db, provided that the two sounds are exactly in phase. If, on the other hand, the sounds are not in phase, then the overall SPL would be increased 3 db—thus 90 db + 90 db = 93 db.

Instruments for measuring sound are called sound-level meters and analyzers. The sound-level meter consists of a microphone, an amplifier, and an indicator. The meters respond to frequencies between 20 to 20,000 HZ. Current instruments are designed to meet specifications established by the United States of America Standards Institute (USASI). Most sound-level meters are equipped with three electrical weighting or filter networks A, B, and C, which enable the instrument to approximate the response of the ear at sound-pressure levels about 40, 70, and 100 db. Figure 3 represents the approximate weighting characteristics for the A, B, and C networks.

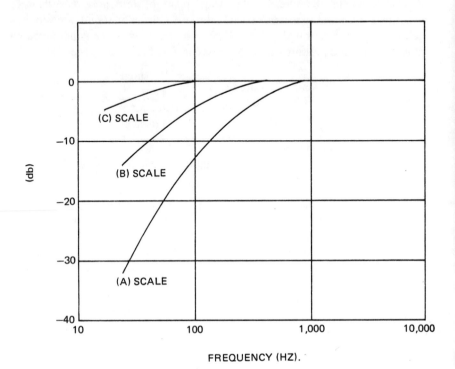

FREQUENCY (HZ).

Figure 3. Weighting characteristics for sound-pressure-level measurements. Most sound-level meters are equipped with three electrical weighting or filter networks (A, B, and C), which enable the instrument to approximate the response of the ear at different sound-pressure levels.

Because the various networks cut out certain portions of the lower frequencies, it is important that the network utilized for obtaining an SPL measurement be part of the designation for that measurement—for example, 78 dbA, 78 dbB, or 78 dbC. If the network is not shown, then it must be assumed that the measurement was made utilizing the "C" scale. This network aspect can be confusing, since a noise source may have sound-pressure-level readings of 75 dbA and 95 dbC, while another source may have readings of 75 dbA and 80 dbC. If we compare these two sources by their "A" scale readings, it might be assumed that they are of equal intensities. On the other hand, their "C" scale readings are quite different.[1] It is, therefore, important that these facts be kept in mind when attempting to compare intensities of different sources.

A number of sound-measuring meters also contain frequency analyzers, which are capable of determining intensities with discrete frequency ranges. The most common type of frequency-band analyzer permits analysis of frequency bands one octave in width.

Excessive exposure of humans to noise can produce both physical and psychological manifestations. The initial symptoms of noise exposure below the threshold of pain are usually discomfort, headache, and temporary hearing loss. If the exposure is allowed to continue over a period of years, gradual permanent hearing impairment may develop. During the youthful years—up to 30—noise-induced damage is rarely permanent, with the effects being sufficiently mild to be reversible.

Other physiological effects besides hearing impairment have been reported. Certain noises may produce alterations in respiration, circulation, basal metabolic rate, and muscle tension. Workers exposed to noise have complained of irritability and sleeping disturbances. Reactions may be manifested by nausea, vomiting, and disturbances of equilibrium. Noise-exposed workers have also been subject to chronic gastritis. Increases in peripheral vascular resistance and decreases in arterial blood flow along with diminution in salivary gland and gastric secretions may also result. Foreign studies have reported an increased incidence of cardiovascular ailments in workmen routinely exposed to high levels of industrial noise. In some cases, a fatal effect has been ascribed to highly intense jet plane noise.

Equally as important and very likely more important than the physical effects are the possible psychological effects. Psychological reactions, similar to physical responses, involve a multiplicity of factors which vary with the characteristics of the sound—its intensity, frequency, intermittency—as well as the inappropriateness of the stimulus, interference with speech communications, and the unexpectedness of the noise. The type of noise, rather than the intensity, is usually the deciding factor in influencing emotional reactions. A sudden scream, a grating piece of chalk, and a dripping faucet—all involve different yet characteristic emotional responses. Unfortunately, our knowledge has not yet reached the point where the complaint threshold associated with a given noise stimulus can be predicted with any degree of reliability; the variations of human responses are simply too great. Furthermore, we are totally

---

[1] The "C" network represents essentially a flat response between 50 to 10,000 HZ while the "A" network filters out a significant portion of the intensity below 500 HZ. It can be concluded that the source represented by the 95 dbC reading contains much more of its energy in the frequencies below 500 HZ than the source represented by the 80 dbC reading. Thus the frequency spectra of the two sources will be different.

ignorant of the overall long-term effects to our physical and psychological well-being from these continued annoyances.

Humans develop hearing loss with aging. Figure 4 is a summary of five studies involving hearing loss with age in men. In the past the gradual degradation of the hearing ability of the general population was thought to be strictly due to the aging process. A hearing study conducted among one African tribe indicates that the tribal elders suffered much less hearing loss than did their modern urban contemporaries. These tribesmen lived in an atmosphere of virtual silence. On the other hand, a similar investigation was conducted among an order of cloistered nuns whose exposure to urban noises was limited. The hearing acuity of this group of women was the same as, and in some instances less than, that of a comparable population. Obviously, the question of the influence of aging on hearing loss has not been entirely settled.

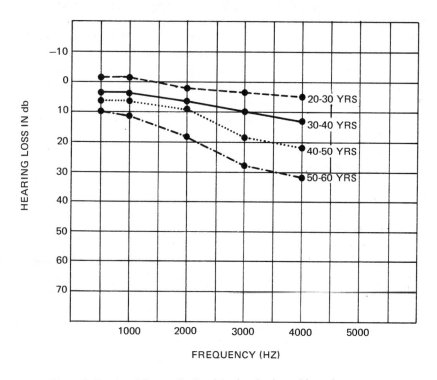

Figure 4. Results of five studies involving hearing loss with age in men.

A significant portion of our population has, in the past, been exposed to industrial noise in addition to urban noise. Hearing surveys (Figure 5) have, in fact, shown that hearing sensitivity is poorer in factory workers and other

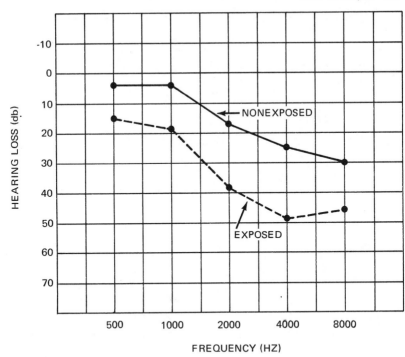

Figure 5. Hearing losses by a group exposed to industrial noise (90-100 db) for an average
· period of 26 years exceeded those by a nonexposed group.

industrial groups than in a population with a minimal occupational exposure. An
example of some noise levels associated with industrial operations are shown in
Figures 6 and 7. It should be noted that the risk curves are higher in the lower
frequencies, implying that the lower frequencies are less damaging than are the
higher frequencies. It is significant, however, that industry has made rapid strides
by the use of noise control techniques and hearing protection in its attempts to
minimize this problem.

Noise levels in urban communities are on the rise. The causes are many,
including expanding transportation and industry, population density, and
increased construction. One of the most critical aspects of the urban noise
problem involves the rapidly expanding transportation system, both highway
and air travel. There are, at present, in excess of 100,000,000 vehicles on our
highways, and the number of new vehicles increases every year. The problem is
magnified by the tremendous increase in freeway systems, where both tire design
and roadway composition contribute to noise output.

A few years ago, in a medium-size community, a thoroughfare was located
adjacent to an office building which had formally been situated on a dead-end

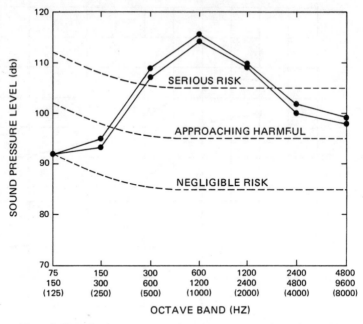

Figure 6. Noise levels associated with a planer, two feet from the machine.

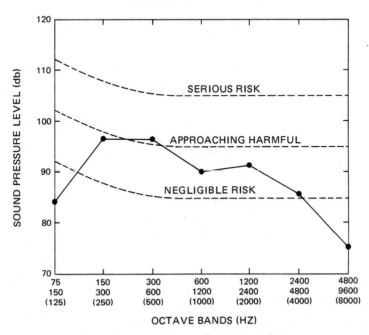

Figure 7. Noise levels from a Presto-log machine.

street. Following this roadway addition, noise levels within the building reached intensities as high as 95 dbC. (See the table.) Levels on the street corner reached 105 dbC. As a result of the noise, many tenants were forced to move.

NOISE LEVELS IN OFFICE BUILDING AND STREET ADJACENT TO BUILDING.

LOCATION	OVERALL SPL (dbC)
Second floor office	
Office "A" windows open	
Background—no traffic	58- 62
Light traffic	64- 72
Logging truck—empty	64- 80
Logging truck—loaded	95
Dump truck	84
Motorcycle	90- 94
Office "A" windows closed	
Background—no traffic	48- 58
Logging truck—loaded	80- 92
Outdoors—front of main entrance—no traffic	64- 68
Logging truck—loaded	100-104-110
Dump truck—loaded	100-102-105
Light traffic	80- 82
1949 sedan	90
Pick-up truck	86
Transit bus	87- 90
Motorcycle	90- 94

In 1968 noise measurements were made in schoolrooms where student hearing screening tests were performed. Those schools located close to busy streets, freeways, and airports experienced noise levels 10 to 15 db above the levels in the other schools. Recently, continuous noise monitoring was accomplished in a school located immediately adjacent to a freeway. During the school day, background noise intensities in an empty classroom facing the freeway averaged between 70 to 74 dbC with maximum levels reaching 92 dbC.

The problem of aircraft noise exists at every major airport in the world. Despite the attempts to limit jet engine noise, this problem will undoubtedly get more severe before adequate controls are promulgated. To the many persons clustered in homes and apartment buildings below or near the flight paths, life can be almost unbearable. E. Thomas Burnard, executive vice president of the Airport Operators Council International states:

Aviation is still a fast growing industry in the U.S. In 1960 only 16 airports serviced jets; today there are 150 airports that receive jets. It is estimated that nearly 350 airports will service jets in 1970 and more than 500 airports will service jets by 1975.

Furthermore, Mr. Burnard, in a statement before the House Subcommittee on Transportation and Aeronautics, reported the following figures for aircraft and aircraft movements.

Year	Jet Air	Aircraft Movements (millions)
1960	224 (turbojets)	26
1966	896	47.8
1974	2240	95.6

The sonic boom controversy presents some very interesting aspects. A Special Study Group on Noise and Sonic Boom in Relation to Man reports that although the sonic boom from an SST would not be harmful to the human ear and although it has not been demonstrated that "startle" responses to the boom would have significant, harmful, psychological effects, it appears that the psychological, sociological, and political reactions of millions of people to the sonic-boom environment from the SST will be extremely adverse and may be of significant magnitude and prevalence to cause partial, if not complete, curtailment of the overland operation of an SST.

This study group indicated that the issues may be clarified through the following questions:

1. Can people "pay" physiologically and mentally the price of being exposed to from one to fifty booms per day from SST?
2. Should people "pay" the price of annoyance and discomfort from being exposed to the booms from a commercial SST?
3. Will the society of the United States "pay" the price of annoyance and discomfort from being exposed to the booms from a commercial SST?

Even in and around the home individuals are exposed to relatively high levels of noise. Responsibility for this assault rests with equipment and machinery including home workshop machines, TVs, radios, hi-fis, food mixers, air conditioners, washers, heating systems, vacuum cleaners, lawn mowers, etc. Noise levels at home may reach 100 db and even higher.

Measurements made by the author during a rock and roll dance reached a maximum of 122 dbC with the average intensity exceeding 104 dbC. A Florida physician concerned about his teenaged daughter's difficulty in hearing, after attending a dance, selected a group of 10 teen-agers and tested their hearing an hour before a dance and again immediately after the dance. All suffered significant temporary hearing impairment, with the greatest impairment being in the high frequency range.

One can conclude that man is exposed to noise from many sources and that all of these sources contribute to the potential damaging effects. The question most often posed is: What can we do about noise? Here we have some answers via technology but many others that take us into the area of value judgments and considerations that are political, economic, or sociological in nature.

The recent interest in operational airport and aircraft noise and the future advent of supersonic transports, with the resulting sonic booms, has prompted a good deal of public attention to the problem of urban noise. As a consequence, there has been an increasing demand for legislation to combat excessive noise. In general, two types of laws have been used in attempts to control noise: nuisance laws and performance zoning codes. Nuisance laws are intended primarily to restrict annoying or unpleasant noise sources which are neither easily measured nor controlled by physical means. The most frequent forms use time limits to prohibit operation or the phrase "loud and annoying to persons of normal sensibilities." In many cases, the action is to prove that the complainer possesses other than normal sensibilities, which may be true or untrue.

Performance zoning codes typically specify the maximum allowable noise at a fixed point and provide relief by specifying limits for noise emitted from various activities. Nominally, these laws are proposed for promoting the public's health, safety, and general welfare while conserving property values and encouraging the most appropriate land use. Both nuisance laws and zoning codes have been used in a number of places in the United States. A review of most of these codes and laws indicates that they are usually ineffective or unenforceable. In either event, this approach has not proved realistic in controlling urban noise, at least at the level I consider desirable.

Many common sources of noise are not amenable to control by these methods. The automotive vehicle, a major source of community pollution including noise, requires special attention as does aircraft noise and noise produced by mechanical devices. Here it becomes imperative that noise control be designed into the basic product. I hope that this can be accomplished voluntarily. If not, then I foresee that federal legislation will be required.

A look at the problem of the barking dog gives some insight into our attempts to control noise sources. Each year numerous complaints are registered because of noisy dogs. According to one local Humane Society, the barking dog and its relation as a public nuisance have long plagued the Humane Society and law-enforcement agencies. Existing laws tend to state that a barking dog may be a nuisance under certain conditions. No known law adequately defines a nuisance as it applies to the barking dog. The courts generally feel that a barking dog can only become a public nuisance if the following factors are part of the problem:

1. The dog must bark or howl.
2. The barking must be excessive.
3. The dog must annoy more than one individual in different households.

4. It must be at a time generally conceded that quiet should reign throughout the neighborhood.

When the Humane Society receives a complaint regarding a barking dog, a letter is sent to the owner informing him that his neighbors have complained and requesting that the nuisance be abated. If the dog owner refuses to comply, the complainants may, with the assistance of two others not of the same household and so affected, register their complaint at the "In Person Complaint Department" in the public safety building. This department may authorize court action.

There appears, however, to be some reluctance on the part of the judiciary to levy "stiff" fines on individuals whose animals have created a nuisance. It has been put forth by some that the way to solve the problem is for the judge to confiscate the animal. However, legally, this tends to be impossible as the animal is considered personal property. Most judges would not have the right to confiscate personal property from an individual as the result of a misdemeanor. It has been suggested that perhaps one way to solve the problem would be to issue a permit to keep the dog, rather than a license. Then, if the dog becomes a public nuisance, the "permit" could be revoked, thereby forcing the owner to remove the animal. Such a procedure would probably be acceptable but would still necessitate legal action.

As you can well imagine, noise pollution control is an extremely complicated endeavor involving numerous variables and factors, many of which are still unknown. Much has been gained from past studies involving aircraft and industrial noise as well as viewpoints from other countries. With the possible exception of aircraft and vehicular noise, no set of maximum noise levels has as yet been adequately validated for use in community regulations. Control of community noise must be recognized and accepted as a major factor in urban planning and development. For this to be accomplished, it would be necessary to establish uniform standards and criteria for evaluating and controlling noise. Because noise is both a local and an area-wide problem, it seems to me that we will have to take the following steps: Appropriate local, state, and federal legislation must be forthcoming in order to support and effect compliance with standards; the manufacturers of mechanical equipment for all phases of use, domestic and industrial, must be made aware of the need to produce quieter equipment; construction codes must also recognize the need for acoustic treatment in homes and buildings.

A major effort will be required to solve the noise-abatement problem. It will be mandatory that many facets of our society—private, industrial, governmental, educational, and technical—assume greater responsibility in the quest for a quieter city. The only question now is . . . are we ready for the challenge? If we are not, then there is one consoling fact . . . as you the reader grow older, you will be disturbed less by noise . . . you will, of course, hear less.

BIBLIOGRAPHY

1. "Aircraft Noise." *Environmental Science and Technology* 1: 976-83; December 1967.
2. Blazier, W. "Criteria for Control of Community Noise." *Sound and Vibration* 2: 11-15; May 1968.
3. _____. "Sonic Boom in Relation to Man." *Scientist and Citizen* 10: 223-229; November 1968.
4. Cohen, A. "Industrial and Community Noise Problems and Legal Efforts at Control." *Journal of Environmental Health* 30: 516-24; March-April 1968.
5. _____. "Location-Design Noise Control of Transportation Systems." United States Department of Health, Education and Welfare, Washington, D.C. January 1967.
6. _____. and R. Scherger. "Correlation of Objectionability Ratings of Noise with Proposed Noise Annoyance Measures." United States Department of Health, Education and Welfare. Washington, D.C. May 1964.
7. *Industrial Noise Manual.* American Industrial Hygiene Association. Detroit, Michigan. 1966. Second Edition.

Radiation

INTRODUCTION

Radiation, properly utilized, is instrumental in improving human health and well-being. The application of x-ray and radioisotopes in clinical diagnosis and therapy; radioisotopes in industry (for measuring, testing and processing); electric power generation; microwave cooking equipment; and lasers (in science, industry and medicine) are just a few examples of beneficial application of radiation.

Exposure to radiation can result in biological damage which may not be immediately apparent. The damage manifests itself in various ways and the timetable of effects-versus-exposure varies widely depending upon the type of radiation, the duration and magnitude of exposure, and portion of the biological system exposed. There are delayed somatic effects such as leukemia, reduced life span, precancerous lesions, and neoplasms which do not appear for years following an acute or a long-term chronic exposure; and there are also those genetic effects (mutations affecting progeny of irradiated persons) which do not become apparent for many generations.

In 1959, the Federal Radiation Coucil (FRC) was formed in the United States to provide a federal policy on human exposure to ionizing radiation. FRC adopted the position that any radiation exposure of the population involves some risk; the magnitude increasing with the exposure. Thus, FRC accepted, for standards setting purposes, the linear or non-threshold concept of the biological effects of ionizing radiation from firm evidence of the effects of high dose and the lack of evidence that low dosages do not produce biological effects. The principal mission of the public and private organizations interested in radiation protection is to minimize exposure of the general population to unnecessary ionizing and non-ionizing radiation from all controllable sources.

Excerpts from *Environmental Health Planning,* U.S. Department of Health, Education and Welfare, Public Health Service Publication 2120, Bureau of Community Environmental Management, 1971.

PROBLEM DEFINITION

Sound program development requires that radiological health problems be defined and their magnitude determined. The public health significance of any specific source of radiation is related to (a) number of sources in use, (b) anticipated growth rate, (c) population at risk, (d) relative toxicity, and (e) length of exposure. The public health significance of any particular source of radiation must also consider the source in relation to the other radiation sources of all types within the environment. Problem identification is necessary to permit rational administrative and functional planning (planning staff requirement, financial needs, instrumentation and laboratory requirements, etc.). Examples of problem areas include:

1. Electronic devices capable of producing radiation which is incidental to their use or which may emit radiation by design. These include but are not limited to, devices used for clinical diagnosis and therapy, educational purposes, commerce and industry and devices used in the home such as television receivers and microwave ovens.

2. Radioactive materials of all types used largely for clinical, industrial and educational purposes.

3. Possible effect on the population and the environment from exposure by an actual or potential discharge of radioactive wastes from nuclear-fueled electric power generating plants and nuclear fuel reprocessing plants, the peaceful uses of nuclear explosives and radioactive material disposal activities.

It is necessary to estimate the number and growth potential of the various radiation sources in order to evaluate the present and anticipated magnitude of public health problems associated with the defined radiation source.

Data Collection

Users of by-product, source, and limited quantities of special nuclear material within a state can be located from licensing information available from AEC or an "Agreement State." Information relating to other sources of radiation including x-ray equipment and radium may be obtained from state health departments, professional organizations, industrial groups, manufacturers, and distributors. Educational institutions can supply data regarding research equipment such as particle accelerators, electron microscopes, lasers, etc. Various state agencies can provide information on power reactors, mining and processing of source material, and waste disposal sites. For reasons of planning and development, radiation sources should be categorized by type of use and a method devised to indicate the number and location of such sources. In defining the problem, there may be more than one element. For example, in a medical and dental x-ray program (1) facilities and equipment should not cause unnecessary exposure, (2) techniques for using equipment should emphasize obtaining optimum clinical results with minimum radiation exposure of patient and operator, and (3) judgments regarding need for specific x-ray examinations or treatments should be made with appropriate consideration of the potential hazards of radiation exposure as well as of the clinical indications of the procedure. Thus, in developing objectives and the plan of action, there may be several lines of approach to remedy the situation.

Understanding the Atom

As you read these lines, your body is under bombardment by streams of radiation pouring in from outer space—the cosmic rays. Other forms of radiation from radioactive atoms in the earth itself add to the intensity of the attack; some of these may be emanating from the walls of the room in which you are sitting, in fact they probably are. Within your body itself, particularly in the bones, radioactive substances are pouring out particles that penetrate the living tissue. If all of these particles can be likened to bullets, then your body is being riddled with machine-gun fire from all angles at all times, day and night.

> Radioactivity is a characteristic of an atom that discharges radiation.
> Radiation is a transfer of energy.
> Radiation is not necessarily radioactive in origin.
> Any atoms having the same number of protons and electrons are isotopes.

Yet you are still alive, and presumably none the worse for it. Natural radioactivity has not prevented life from evolving on earth, nor man as a species from developing his position of preeminence. From this it may be assumed that irradiation of the magnitude normally encountered in our environment cannot do us any great harm. As the scientists say, we are "in biological equilibrium" with this phenomenon. And since natural radiation in certain parts of the world is known to be several times the average without apparently causing ill effects, it is reasonable to conclude that man may expose himself to additional artificial radiation of about the same magnitude as the average background radiation without any harmful consequences. In other words, high natural radiation provides a safety mark, showing us that we can take at least that much radiation.

Radiation thus forms a permanent part of our environment, but it is only recently that we have begun to understand what it is all about.

Reprinted by permission from *World Health,* January 1969.

Not So Wild A Dream

Man has been looking for a way to change the structure of things for a long time. During the Middle Ages, the fires of alchemists' stoves showed that the search to transmute metals was going on. It was never to succeed but the very failures laid the base of modern chemistry. Later investigations showed that there were about ninety substances that could neither be broken into simpler ones nor synthesized from others already known. They were called the elements. This meant abandonment of the search for a philosopher's stone to change one element into another. The nineteenth century was sure that in this respect the end of the line had been reached since the unchangeable foundations of nature were known.

> The Three R's.
> The potency of radiation in all forms is measured in three ways.
> The **rontgen** gives the amount of radiation absorbed in air at a given point. The **rad** gives the amount of radioactive energy actually held in a gram of any material. The **rem** indicates the degree of potential danger to health, and is the rad multiplied by a given factor of potential danger. The radiation to which the average citizen is exposed is made up almost wholly of the fast-moving, highly-penetrating X-rays, gamma rays, and beta rays, where rem and rad are equal. (See section on danger for tolerable levels of radiation to man.)

A cluster of discoveries during the last decade of the nineteenth century were to start a revolution in knowledge which is still going on and were to lead to the alchemist's dream being realized in an unexpected way.

Rontgen was the first to use X-rays in order to study bone structure that was previously invisible. As early as the first year of Rontgen-ray use, reports began to come in about "changes of the skin similar to the effects of sunburn" which later proved to be various forms of radiation damage. Thus side by side with progress, a new series of dangers was being revealed. However, the determination and selfless devotion of such people as Rontgen and the Curies, showed that radiation could be used for man's advantage. There is no doubt that the more we know about the elements which compose our world the better we will be able to use them to good purpose.

The Basic Facts

All tangible things around us—the chair we sit in, the pencil in our hands, and we ourselves—are combinations of elements; each of these has certain physical and chemical properties. The smallest particle of an element is called the "atom."

The atoms themselves are not little building blocks but are more like tiny solar systems in which a nucleus consisting of neutrons and protons has a number of electrons circling around it. Each atom of the same element has the same number of protons in its nucleus and electrons in orbit; these determine the chemical properties of the element. However, two atoms of the same element may have an identical number of protons and electrons but a different number of neutrons. Thus one nucleus will be heavier, that is to say contain more neutrons, than another.

Doing What Comes Naturally

When the number of protons and neutrons becomes too great the nucleus begins to break down, or rather to unload protons and neutrons. This may be inherent in some forms of unstable matter such as uranium, or else be induced artificially. In either case, this unloading or emission of radiation in the form of a stream of particles, or rays, is known as radioactivity; the atom emitting the rays is called a radioisotope.

The best known of the naturally radioactive substances are probably radium and uranium, and these are still widely used by man for his own purposes; in a similar way he harnessed other natural sources of energy, for example running water and the wind. Like the rivers and the wind, these radioactive substances are always there. They can be used, they can be diverted or obstructed to some extent, but they cannot be obliterated.

Natural radiation, like many other natural phenomena, is not totally harmless. The point is rather that life flourishes notwithstanding, so that the damage done to the sum of mankind is almost negligible. It has been estimated, for example, that natural radiation accounts for about 10 percent of the incidence of leukemia, a comparatively rare disease in which the white blood corpuscles multiply at the expense of the red (see World Health, June '68), causing glandular trouble and finally, in time, death. From this it is possible to calculate the likely increase in leukemia resulting from background radiation at various levels, if one assumes that there is a simple arithmetical relationship between the two—double the radiation, double the number of cases attributable to this cause.

This assumption is made because at present we have no means of knowing why a particular person exposed to minute doses of radioactive matter shows ill effects while tens of thousands, if not millions, of individuals in the same environment show none. For practical purposes we can only assume that it is a question of chance, and that the chances of a particular person being the unlucky one are remote. Therefore, the only way to safeguard the unknown individual who might be struck down some day is to protect the entire community. Control of the radiation level is thus a public health responsibility if ever there was one.

Apart from the way in which it is produced, there is nothing really "artificial" about artificial radiation to distinguish it from natural radiation.

Whereas uranium, for example, has been emitting radiation of its own accord for millions of years, man has only recently learned, through the use of electricity or by splitting the atom, to set this process going. Scientists can now upset the balance of almost all known atoms, by adding a neutron to the nucleus and so causing a discharge of particles, thus making the atom radioactive. However, whether these "live" atoms are artificially triggered off or derived from naturally radioactive materials, they discharge the same radiation and for practical purposes their uses in medicine and industry are the same. What is important, therefore, is not the origin of the process but rather the type and quantity of radiation.

The ABC of ABG

There are three kinds of radiation known as alpha particles, beta particles, and gamma rays, each of which has certain advantages and drawbacks. Some rays are more potent in their biological effects than others; alpha particles, for example, are ten times as harmful as X-rays, beta particles or gamma rays. Alpha particles, luckily, have little penetrating force—generally speaking they cannot penetrate even this sheet of paper; hence they do not constitute a considerable outside health risk to the body. On the other hand, they are quite dangerous if radioactive substance has entered the body (by inhalation or through a wound). Thus workers handling radioactive substances in industry require suitable protection.

Gamma rays are deep-penetrating radiations, similar to X-rays, which are electromagnetic waves, not streams of physical particles. In industry, gamma rays are in fact often used for the same purpose as X-rays, by means of a small portable apparatus loaded with a capsule of radioactive matter. These instruments are much handier than X-ray installations—many of them are no bigger than a football—but X-rays can be switched off, while the radioactive substance in such capsules never ceases to emit potentially harmful rays, both beta and gamma. This illustrates that the origin of the rays does not alter their effects, but the technique for producing them can be an important factor in occupational safety.

The Dangerous Atom

Robert Plant

Medical men divide the ill effects of radiation into three categories. First, there is the evident risk of more or less immediate injury, the *somatic* or bodily effects. Second, there are the delayed effects, in extreme cases not discernible for as long as 50 years after exposure; these might be termed the *delayed somatic* effects. Finally, there are the *genetic effects,* which do not affect us directly but appear in our progeny.

In the main, the somatic effects are those which persons exposed in medicine and industry may suffer. Localized somatic symptoms were observed as early as 1896, one year after the discovery of X-rays—reddening of the exposed areas, wounds looking like burns, ulceration of the skin. Later, general symptoms, such as lassitude, nausea and general weakness were noticed. By 1903, it had been demonstrated experimentally on animals that radiation retarded bone growth, and by 1905 that it affected the blood. A case where a human foetus was exposed by mistake during X-ray examination of the mother showed that the whole growth and development of a child can be greatly handicapped. The risk of injury is particularly serious to the more delicate tissues of the body, such as the eyes, the genitals, the bloodforming organs and growing glands, and the female breast.

The somatic symptoms may not appear for some time. The normal latent period is a matter of weeks, but the damage begins with radiation and may take time to build up to a clinical condition. A malignant growth, for example, that does not become manifest for perhaps five years after the exposure, should not be confused with a delayed somatic injury, in which the deterioration does not, as far as can be determined, make a start until long after the event.

For somatic injury a certain minimum dose seems to be required, a threshold which may be approached but not passed with safety. A dose of 25 to 50 roentgens to the whole body was found to affect the white blood corpuscles and to produce mild lassitude and softening of the muscles. The evidence of radiation accidents over the years has shown that 400 to 500 roentgens on the whole body are fatal in about 50 percent of cases, and 600 to 700 in practically every case. This knowledge makes it relatively simple, in principle, to protect the

Reprinted by permission from *World Health,* January 1969.

citizen from the risk of somatic radiation injury—such injury can only be the result of negligence, ignorance or accident. The maximum permitted dose in the ILO code for radiation workers, averaged out for several years, amounts to about 100 millirems per week.

More Mysterious

Delayed somatic injury is a more mysterious phenonmenon. Years after the bombing of Hiroshima and Nagasaki, it was found that the number of leukemia cases reported in those areas was in proportion to population five to ten times larger than in other parts of Japan. It is always difficult to show a measurable relationship between injury and radiation in delayed somatic cases, because of the long time lag and because other causes may have been at work, but it is now fairly well established that delayed effects are mainly of three kinds: leukemia, malignant tumours, and shortening of life.

In animals, delayed malignant tumours have been induced by comparatively heavy doses, 100 roentgens and more. A direct arithmetical relationship has also been demonstrated between the amount of radiation received by mice and their length of life. This, too, was established by experiments involving fairly high doses, 50 roentgens and over. To obtain reliable information using smaller doses would require testing more animals than is practicable, but if the effects are directly proportional to the amount of radiation received, down to the lowest levels—in other words, if there is no threshold—then it can be calculated that a dose of one roentgen on the whole body would reduce the average expectation of a man's life by about three days. From this it is not difficult to work out the length of time by which the life would be shortened of, say, an industrial worker exposed regularly to the maximum dose permitted by the ILO code. This being on average 5 rems per year, he might lose 15 days of life for every year he worked. A radiologist receiving the maximum permitted dose in hospitals—which is at the same level of about 5 rems per year—over a working career of 40 years might lose one-and-a-half years of life.

Nobody is likely to be exposed to the maximum permitted dose many years of his working life, and the assumptions on which these calculations are made are of course speculative, to say the least. They are, however, the assumptions on which we have to work at the present time. What is certain is that radiation exposure can shorten life, and does so appreciably. This has nothing to do with discernible injury. We just don't live as long.

Mutations

Genetic effects should not be confused with injury to the sex organs or injury to an unborn baby; strictly speaking, these are somatic effects. Genetic effects proper are revealed only in future generations. They are the result of damage to the chromosomes. Every human cell contains 46 chromosomes, 23 inherited from the mother and 23 from the father, and each chromosome contains hundreds of thousands of *genes,* by which the characteristics of the species and indeed of different individuals are transmitted to the offspring. Radiation injury can take two forms, named by medical men *chromosome mutations* and *point mutations.* The former involve damage to the whole chromosome and can be detected by a microscope; the latter leave the chromosome alive but touch the genes.

Chromosome mutations require a certain minimum dose—in other words, there is a threshold—and the chromosomes occasionally recover. Generally, they entail the death of the cell to which they belong. If that cells finds its way into the reproductive process, obviously the possibilities of fertilization are reduced. Hence there is a connection between chromosome mutation and sterility. It is a matter of chance, and of pretty remote chance in the average individual, but in a population of millions somebody will be unlucky in the draw.

To the layman, the most sinister of all radiation effects is point mutation. The cell is not killed, life can still be transmitted, but the offspring may be malformed in ways we cannot foresee. Here there is apparently no threshold; a single "hit" by a radioactive ray can cause the damage, which of itself is too slight even to be visible under the microscope. The only comfort is that the probabilities involved are remote. First, there is the chance of a particular person sustaining the injury. Then there is the chance of the cell containing the chromosome with the damaged genes finding its way into the reproductive process. Finally, it is necessary for both parents to have sustained the injury for the mutation to be passed on. So high are the odds against, that we are not likely to see the consequences in our lifetime. Professor Walter Seelentag of WHO says: "With certain qualifications, an increase in the mutation rate after irradiation will probably be manifest only after many generations."

At first, this seems rather consoling, but only at first. The thought that by our complacent acceptance of the benefits of radiation we may be causing some child to be born malformed, long after we have lived out our natural lives and are resting in our graves, must surely appall any person of imagination and conscience. One is forced to echo Shakespeare's Hamlet, speaking four centuries ago: "The dread of something after death . . . must give us pause."

The Burden Today

Cosmic rays are weakened as they pass through the atmosphere, but at ordinary living altitudes their impact is about 35 millirems a year. Terrestrial radiation, emananting from the earth's crust, varies greatly: in Kerala, in India, for example, where there are rock formations containing uranium, it can be as high as 1000 millirads a year. At the other extreme, parts of Germany with mainly basalt formations have recorded as little as 14 millirads a year and parts of England where limestone predominates, 26 millirads. The average is about 50. Natural radiations from other sources, such as the air around us, add another 20 or so. This radiation originates in the earth but hits us at second hand, so to speak. Internal radiation, from radioactive matter in the body, is thought to inflict about 25 millirads a year on the body as a whole but may be as high as 70 or 80 in the bone marrow. All in all, it is estimated that the total natural radiation to which the average person is subjected comes to about 175 millirems a year.

On balance, the protection afforded by buildings is offset by radiation from the structure itself. Most materials act as partial shields, but they also contain traces of radioactive elements; they parry and thrust at the same time. Research in Sweden, for example, revealed that radiation inside wooden houses was 50 millirads a year, inside brick houses 104 millirads a year and inside slate concrete houses, 171 millirads, while in the streets of Stockholm 85 millirads a year was recorded.

Some everyday appliances are radioactive. Television tubes emit X-rays, but these are too feeble to travel far and are almost completely absorbed in the set. Shoe fitting fluoroscopes were found to impose a considerable load, in one case as high as 10 roentgens a year on a child's foot through repeated use, but these instruments are now employed with greater caution and the effect is slight. Until a few years ago in a European country where research was conducted, luminous wristwatches were found to be inflicting a local dose to the skin ranging from 1.3 to 30 roentgens a year. This weakened as it traveled through the body, but the genetic exposure—the irradiation of the sex organs—still worked out at an average per person over the whole population of 2.5 millirads a year. The radium formerly used to luminize the dials of watches and clocks has now been superseded by less dangerous substances, from which the dose to the body as a whole is negligible. In general it may be said that radiation from everyday appliances is at present too small to be important. But, like all the uses of radiation, it is growing.

Medical uses of radiation amounted in 1963 in a typical industrialized country, Germany (F.R.), to an average of 23.5 millirems for every member of the population, of which 22 millirems were received by the patients and 1.5 by the staff. Of course these are average figures meaning that doses received may be much higher or lower per person according to the case. Staff in industry and research, in this country, accounted for less than a millirem—0.7 to be exact—per member of the population, and various other sources added 2.5 millirems. Fallout amounted to 33 millirems per capita bringing the total for 1963 to almost 60 millirems.

A Need for Better Technique

At this point, the reader may protest that the dose received by many individuals, particularly those working in medicine and industry, must have been very much higher than the average, and this of course is true. The necessity of safeguarding persons where there is a high risk of exposure is everywhere recognized. Techniques for limiting the exposure of hospital patients to the practical minimum and avoiding irradiation of the sex glands are also obviously important and can in many cases be improved. The figures show that in Britain, for example, a country with generally high standards, the factor the experts call the "genetically significant dose" would be reduced by 80 percent if techniques in all hospitals were raised to the level of the best. The situation in other countries is doubtlessly similar. It is a matter of directing the rays carefully to the areas under examination and, if necessary, of shielding the vital parts. To assess the radiation load on the people as a whole, however, which is the public health authority's concern, these local concentrations have to be worked into the national average. Only in this way can some measurement be attempted of the overall danger, particularly where casualties may be a matter of chance. The urgent thing for the public health expert is to keep within bounds—if he can—the total volume of irradiation in the community.

The burden from radioactive fallout is really in a category by itself. Being man made, it is certainly artificial radiation, but it is not produced voluntarily by most of the communities on which it descends. It consists of radioactive particles released into the atmosphere by an atomic explosion, floating down to earth for some years afterwards. Because of the height to which the particles are driven and the effect of air currents, it is distributed fairly evenly over the whole human race. It is falling on you now. It subsides in time, but, so long as above-ground tests of nuclear weapons continue, the supply is replenished. Measurements made in 1963 in Germany, (F.R.), a country where there had been no explosions, showed that a dose of 33 millirems per person was received from this source—representing more than half of the 60 millirems attributed to all artificial radioactivity and radiation. Fallout is indeed practically the only man-made background radiation to which the man in the street is exposed at present. Medical and industrial radiation, after all, are kept in their place.

Only the Beginning . . . .

Very broadly, it may be said that artificial radiation from all sources does not yet exceed the natural product. So far, not too bad. But we are only at the beginning.

Scientists and industrialists, if not soldiers, are bound to make increasing use of this extraordinary force which they can now manipulate but not control. Many of the artificial uses of ionizing rays benefit man, and under proper conditions add only small doses of radioactivity to our environment. These doses add up, however; each use is developed without reference to the others, the total grows . . . How far dare we let this process go?

The ordinary man knows that he must accept the dangers of his natural environment, but he sees no reason why he should endure hazards created by the human will, unless the benefit greatly exceeds the harm. He is at the mercy of a danger that is at the same time universal and insidious: it respects no frontiers, and man has no natural sense by which to know its presence. He cannot see it, he cannot smell it, he cannot taste it, he cannot hear it, he cannot touch it. He only knows it is always there, the invisible peril. He is an innocent in the hands of the experts.

Surely he is entitled to ask that the process be brought under control before it is too late. He asks this, moreover, not only in his own name. He asks it on behalf of a child without a name, not to be born perhaps for a hundred years, who may be the victim of his indifference.

MAN MOST VULNERABLE

Vulnerability to radioactivity is illustrated in the table on page 129 giving approximate orders of magnitude. Doses of 600 to 700 rads are usually fatal for man, one of the most vulnerable of living organisms. Plant germination can be stopped by doses of about 10,000 rads. To destroy insects, higher doses are usually necessary and insects can sometimes survive doses of as much as 40,000 rads. There is some overlapping between the upper limits of radioactivity sufficient to stop plant germination and the lower limits sufficient to kill insects. Destruction of molds results from doses that may vary between 100,000 and 1,000,000 rads. The range between which various forms of molds can resist the destructive effects of radioactivity is considerable.

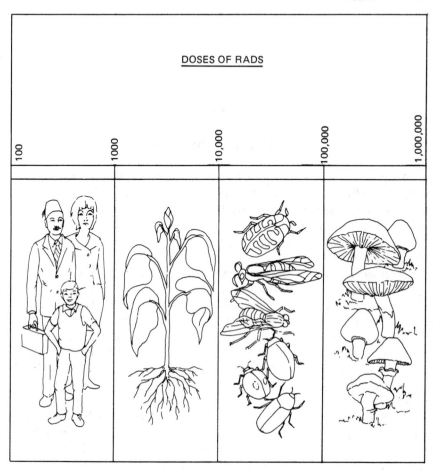

Never Do Harm

Karl Z. Morgan

Medical x-rays save many lives but can also unnecessarily cause the deaths and genetic effects we associate with other forms of radiation. About 95 percent of man-made exposure to radiation in the United States is from medical exposure, and 90 percent of this is from diagnostic x-rays.[1] This exposure could be reduced to one-tenth of its present amount without any loss of the benefits of diagnostic x-rays.

Most of the medical x-ray machines in the United States are owned and operated by nonradiologists (such as physicians and chiropractors) who, in the vast majority of cases, have no education in health physics or radiation protection and no training in the use of x-ray equipment. Fortunately, their x-ray workloads are relatively low, so more than half[2] of the medical diagnostic x-rays in the United States are taken under the supervision (often in absentia) of radiologists. These specialists are trained in the use of such equipment and usually obtain far more useful diagnostic information with less exposure to the patient (there are, of course, exceptions to any such general rule).

To illustrate the desirability of limiting the use of medical diagnostic x-ray equipment to specialists, I call attention to the 1964 U.S. Public Health surveys[3] which indicated that abdominal examinations by radiologists delivered average skin doses of only 490 millirads in comparison with 1,034 millirads delivered in offices of other physicians. (A millirad is one-thousandth of a rad; the rad, "radiation absorbed dose," is the standard unit of measure of radiation exposure.) At present, only the state of California requires education in radiation protection and training in the use of x-rays in the medical schools and questions on the state board examinations on these subjects. Only the states of New York, New Jersey, and California require such training and certification of x-ray technologists. A bill (S. 3973) has been introduced in the Senate by Senator Jennings Randolph (Dem.-West Virginia) which is "to amend the Public Health Services Act to provide for the protection of the public health from unnecessary medical exposure to ionizing radiation." If this bill becomes law, all

Reprinted by permission from *Environment,* 13, No. 1: 28-30 (January/February, 1971.).

states will be required to establish training and certification programs for x-ray technologists. I believe that since a majority of the personnel who use diagnostic x-rays lack the education, training, certification, and motivation in the proper and safe use of ionizing radiation, there is a need for programs which will restrict all use of medical x-rays to those who meet minimum requirements of training in the proper and safe use of this most important medical tool.

The situation with dentists is just as bad. Surveys[3] in the United States have indicated that in more than half of the dental radiograms taken, the x-ray beam covers three or more times the area of the film. This situation persists in most—if not all—countries of the world, in spite of the fact that devices have been developed[4] which may be attached to the end of the long, open-ended cone of the dental x-ray machine to provide precision focusing and reduce the cross-sectional area of the beam to the area of the film.

MEDICAL EXPOSURE HIGHEST

Table 1 summarizes the principal sources of population exposure to ionizing radiation in the United States showing the major role played by medical exposure. Here it is to be observed that the dose from weapons fallout is relatively small and declining steadily. The dose of about 0.6 millirad per year from occupational exposure is quite low, but can be expected to increase considerably in the future due to expansions in the nuclear energy industry and the increasing use of radioisotopes. Radiation from miscellaneous sources undoubtedly will increase because many new types of electronic products added each year to the public market will find their way into research laboratories, industries, hospitals, public schools, and homes. The number of annual medical x-ray examinations in the United States has doubled about every thirteen years[5] and may be increasing at a faster rate due to expansions in Medicare and Medicaid. We cannot afford to permit this increase in the use of ionizing radiation in research, education, medicine, industry, and domestic applications to be an excuse for increasing the average population dose. In this case, I am referring both to the genetically significant dose and the somatic (all tissue other than reproductive cells) dose, and mostly to the low-dose range such as that from x-ray diagnosis.

It is generally believed that the somatic doses of greatest concern are those to red bone marrow which relate to leukemia, those to tissues of the skeleton which are thought to relate to bone tumors, those to tissue of the cental nervous system (CNS) which relate to CNS tumors, those to thyroid and adjacent tissue which relate to thyroid cancer, and those to the body as a whole which are thought to relate to various forms of nonspecific radiation damage resulting in a shortening of the average life expectancy. In this list, I have purposely omitted

TABLE 1

**AVERAGE IONIZING RADIATION EXPOSURE TO
PERSONS LIVING IN THE UNITED STATES**

	Millirems per year	Source*
Medical exposure		
Gonad**dose from diagnosis (1964)	55.0	27
Gonad dose from therapeutic use (1964)	7.0	28
Bone marrow dose from diagnosis (1964)	125.0	29
Thyroid dose from diagnosis (mostly dental) (1964)	1000.0	28
Weapons fallout dose (1968)	2.0***	30
Occupational exposure		
Nuclear energy industry gonad dose (1970)	0.8****	31
All other occupational exposure gonad dose (1966)	0.4	31
Other man-made sources (watches, television, shoe-fitting machines, radioisotope applications, etc.) gonad dose (1966)	0.1	31
Natural background radiation (whole body)	100.0	35

*See the sources listed under Notes at the end of the article.

**Testes and ovaries.

***Gonad and total body dose from cesium-137 estimated to be 1.2 millirems in 1966, 0.68 millirem in 1967, and 0.54 millirem in 1968. The average dose to bone marrow from strontium-90 estimated to be 3.6 millirems in 1966, 2.8 millirems in 1967 and 2.3 millirems in 1968.

****Includes all occupational and environmental exposure from all nuclear energy research and production operations.

the lens of the eye as a critical tissue in reference to the relatively low doses from medical x-ray diagnosis, because there is some evidence that lens cataracts are a threshold type of damage which is not produced in man at doses below about 500 rems. (The rem is a unit roughly equivalent to the rad.) Opacities of various grades are produced at lesser doses. These can be detected and scored by highly skilled observation, and they range in severity all the way from the barely detectable to changes in translucency and refraction that interfere with vision. Perhaps the most disconcerting uncertainty about the low-dose effects of ionizing radiation on the lens of the human eye is the suggestion of a committee of the International Commission for Radiological Protection (ICRP)[6] that senile cataracts may be augmented or accelerated by radiation, perhaps through a synergistic interaction of radiation and age. There are two types of radiation damage—one that varies more or less in straight-line fashion (linearly) with the accumulated dose of ionizing radiation and the other which requires a threshold before it makes its appearance. Radiation sickness (threshold of about 20 rems) and radiation fatalities (threshold of about 300 rems) illustrate the threshold types of damage which should be of no concern to the medical profession except in the case of radiation accidents or, for example, where radiation therapy is used in the treatment of leukemia. Genetic mutations (a doubling dose—the amount of radiation which would double the incidence of mutations—for man assumed to be between 30 to 90 rems) and life shortening (a loss of two and one-half days of life per rem of chronic exposure and thirteen days per rem of short-term exposure) illustrate the types of damage which are thought to relate more or less linearly to the dose. Also, various forms of malignancy such as leukemia, bone tumors, CNS tumors, and thyroid cancer are thought to vary linearly with the accumulated dose. These are the kinds of damage which especially concern us in discussing the need for reduction of unnecessary medical diagnostic exposure and the extreme importance of minimizing the genetic and whole-body dose from all sources of ionizing radiation exposure.

ACCEPTABLE LEVEL

A number of national and international organizations have indicated that the population dose should be kept as low as practicable, and that in any case the total dose should not be more than that which the average person receives from natural background radiation. The ICRP[7] has suggested an absolute upper limit of 5,000 millirems over 30 years (or an average of 170 millirems per year) for this dose exclusive of natural background radiation and medical exposure. In early reports of ICRP,[8] suggestions were made as summarized in Table 2 as to how this 170 millirems per year might be apportioned to various sources of population exposure such as internal and external sources, occupational exposure, exposure of special groups, and a reserve. In its later reports,[7] however, ICRP no longer suggested an apportionment of this dose; rather, it recommended this apportioning be done by appropriate and responsible authorities in each individual country as indicated by local needs and requirements and as "determined by national, economic and social considerations." Some countries have taken the lead and apportioned this 170 millirems per year, but, so far, this apportioning has not been done by any of our national organizations (such as the Federal Radiation Council, the National Council on Radiation Protection and Measurements or the Department of Health, Education and Welfare). This

TABLE 2

**HOW THE GENETIC DOSE TO THE POPULATION
OF 5,000 MILLIREMS OF RADIATION OVER 30 YEARS
MIGHT BE DIVIDED AS SUGGESTED IN 1958 BY THE
INTERNATIONAL COMMISSION FOR RADIOLOGICAL PROTECTION**

Occupational exposure	1,000
Exposure of special groups	500
Reserve	1,500
Nonoccupational—internal exposure	1,500
Nonoccupational—external exposure	500
Total*	5,000

*Exceeds natural background radiation and medical exposure.

might be considered one of the most important tasks to be performed under the Radiation Control for Health and Safety Act of 1968 (PL 90-602). The evaluation of risks versus benefits of medical exposure and the assignment of appropriate upper limits of population exposure from diagnostic and therapeutic doses as well as the allowable dose from all other sources of radiation exposure of the population is a most important responsibility of a number of agencies of our government. Those charged with carrying out this assignment must weigh not only the wonderful benefits of medical applications of x-rays against the serious risks of genetic mutations, leukemia, other malignancies and life shortening, but also the similar benefits and risks from exposure to all sources of radiation exposure. They must weigh the risks of radiation exposure from color television against its entertainment and educational values, the consequences of exposure from the radioactive effluent from nuclear power plants against the advantages of adequate, pure water supplies by desalinization, and home heating, made possible by cheap electrical power from a source causing far less environmental contamination and fewer cases of lung diseases such as emphysema and chronic bronchitis. They must weigh the risks versus the benefits of industrial uses of x-rays which, for example, through industrial radiography help assure that the wings of an airplane are free of internal metallurgical flaws that could otherwise, without x-ray inspection, make air transportation extremely hazardous. Figure 1 illustrates the balancing of risks and benefits from all electromagnetic and particulate radiation received by the total population including future generations. It should be noted, too, that several forms of nonionizing radiation are thought to result in some of the same types of biological damage mentioned above; for example, cataracts and genetic muta- tions are also caused by electromagnetic radiation, and so they must be considered as a part of the total problem.

LOWERING THE DOSE

In the 1967 Congressional hearings[9] in support of PL 90-602, I and a number of other witnesses listed many ways (some 70 altogether) by which medical diagnostic exposure to the population could be reduced to no more than 10 percent of its present level. Further support of the feasibility of such a goal is given by Table 3 which shows that medical diagnostic exposure to the U.S. population is among the highest reported in various advanced countries and by the statement of G. M. Adrian[10] of the United Kingdon, "If all the radiation departments [in the United Kingdom] employed the techniques already in use in 25 percent of the departments in 1958, the population gonad [testes and ovaries] dose from diagnostic radiology would probably be reduced by a factor of about 7." This would correspond to a reduction from the present United Kingdom value of fourteen millirems per year to two millirems per year. A recent report of the U.S. Public Health Service[11] stated, "It was estimated that restriction of the x-ray beam to an area no larger than the film size would result in a reduction of the genetically significant dose from 55 to 19 millirads per person per year." Undoubtedly, such action would reduce the somatic dose to the whole body even more. A number of the other dose-reducing measures could be equally as effective in reducing medical and dental x-ray doses to the patient. On this basis, I believe that a reduction in the United States of the 1964 average medical diagnostic dose from 55 millirems per year to 5 millirems per year does not seem at all unrealistic. In the Congressional hearings[9] in 1967 in support of PL 90-602, I gave some estimates of lives lost per year as a result of radiation damage from medical diagnostic x-rays. These data are reproduced here as Table 4. They are based on the assumption of a linear relationship between dose and effect for these types of damage. For the most part, the assumptions are based on data from reports of the United Nations Scientific Committee on the Effects of Atomic Radiation (UNSCEAR).[12] The genetic deaths are the lethal equiv- alents introduced into the population each year by 55 millirems per year of genetically significant, diagnostic population dose. This number of deaths would occur each year only after a number of years, when equilibrium had been reached. It is to be noted that there is a large spread (2,000 to 26,000) in the estimated number of genetic deaths per year in the United States from diagnostic medical exposure. The lower figure (2,000) corresponds to the lowest estimate of mutations caused by chronic low dose rates of exposure, whereas the larger figure (26,000) corresponds to the higher estimate of mutations caused by high dose rates (greater than 90 rads per minute in the case of mice used in the

TABLE 3

GENETICALLY SIGNIFICANT AND BONE MARROW DOSE TO PEOPLE IN VARIOUS ADVANCED COUNTRIES FROM MEDICAL DIAGNOSTIC X-RAYS

Country	Genetically Significant Dose per Capita (millirems per year)	Source*	Bone Marrow Dose per Capita (millirems per year)	Source*
United States (1964)	55	27	125	34
Germany (Hamburg) (1957-58)	18	32	42	34
Italy (Rome) (1957)	43	32	100	34
Argentina (1950-59)	37	32	85	34
Sweden (1955)	38	27,33	160	34
France (1957-58)	58	32	130	34
Netherlands (Leiden) (1959-60)	6.8	32	15	34
Japan (1958-60)	39	32	90	34
Norway (1958)	10	32	20	34
Denmark (1956)	22	33	50	34
Switerzland (1957)	22	32	50	34
Great Britain (1957-58)	14	32	32	10
UAR (Alexandria, Cairo) (1953-61)	7	32	16	34
New Zealand (1963)	12	27,33	27	34

*See the sources listed under Notes at the end of the article.

studies of Russell).[13] It is not known at present which figure is more applicable to man as a result of diagnostic x-ray exposure, but the high dose rates commonly used in diagnostic x-rays would suggest that the higher estimate of death rate should be used.

I am led to believe that some radiologists would prefer not to be confronted with data such as I have summarized in Table 4 listing the deaths caused each year by medical diagnostic x-rays as estimated when applying the linear hypothesis. Such data, however, are not of my own invention, for these values can be written down by anyone who makes use of the data of the UNSCEAR

TABLE 4

**PRICE TO BE PAID IN DEATHS* PER YEAR IN THE
UNITED STATES AS A CONSEQUENCE OF RADIATION DAMAGE
FROM MEDICAL DIAGNOSTIC EXPOSURE NOW BEING RECEIVED**

Genetic deaths**	2,000 to 26,000
Leukemic deaths	350 to 1,100
Thyroid tumors***from dental x-rays	50 to 400
Thyroid tumors***from mass chest x-rays	5 to 40
Bone tumors***	170 to 550
Life shortening	1,000
Other causes of death	?
Damage other than death	?
Total deaths per year	**3,500 to 29,000+**

*These values are based on the commonly accepted linear hypothesis; namely, 1 rem produces 10 percent the deaths from 10 rem, 0.1 rem produces 1 percent the deaths from 10 rem, etc. They would be the deaths each year at some time in the future assuming the diagnostic dose rates remain constantly at their present values and that the United States population remains static at 200,000,000.

**The number of genetic deaths (or lethal equivalents) is based on the assumption that ultimately each genetic mutation results in a death. A given death may be in the first generation but the vast majority will occur many generations hence. The lower figure is based on the lowest estimate of mutations per rem and on the assumption that human response to diagnostic exposure is similar to that of mice at very low dose rates while the higher figure assumes this response relates to that of mice at high dose rates..

***This assumes none of the tumors are medically treated and each results in a death. The values for thyroid tumors are listed only for children under fifteen years of age and only for dental and mass chest x-rays.

reports[12] and applies them to the U.S. Public Health survey estimates of the average population dose from medical x-rays in the United States. Although the estimates of genetic damage are based[13] on mice experiments, insofar as possible estimates of other damage are based on human experience (extensive surveys of effects of x-ray diagnosis on children exposed before birth, surveys of children whose thyroids were treated with x-rays, bone marrow dose received by ankylosing spondylitis [hardening of the joints between vertebrae] patients, total body dose received by the survivors of atomic bombings of Hiroshima and Nagasaki, etc.). Some persons will object to my assumption of a linear relationship between dose and effect and will say that perhaps at very low doses and dose rates, there may be no such effects or the effects may be greatly reduced. To this, I can only reply that the many scientific committees and the national and international agencies which set the radiation protection standards state that since these effects at high dose rates (where the statistics are good and the probable errors small) seem to relate linearly to the dose, it is prudent that we assume this relationship maintains, also, at lower doses and dose rates.

DIAGNOSTIC RISK

From what has been said above and from the illustrations, we realize that no matter how small the diagnostic exposure, the probability of its inducing serious damage is not zero. The frequency of occurrence of this damage increases with the amount of x-ray dose equivalent (in rem units) and with the equivalent absorbed energy (in gram-rem units) received by the body. There are many studies showing that on a statistical basis diagnostic exposure does result in damage to man. For example, the investigation of the Harvard School of Public Health involved studies[14] of 500,000 infants from 30 United States hospitals. This study indicated that there was about a 30 percent increase in cancer, primarily leukemia and cancer of the central nervous system, in children whose mothers were irradiated during pregnancy. Apparently, the increase took place regardless of successive deliveries, race or sex of the children. Brian MacMahon[15] reported in 1963 that after Alice Stewart's original observations, some twelve studies of the question of the relationship between x-ray exposures of pregnant women (for example, to measure the pelvis) and cancers in children had appeared. He pointed out that although there were positive and negative findings, a combination of data from all of them weighed in accordance with the number of cases studied indicated that mortality from leukemia and other forms of cancer is about 40 percent higher among children exposed to diagnostic x-rays in utero than among children not so exposed. He went on to show that the excess risk over the first ten years of life amounts to about one cancer death per 2,000 children exposed. A study by A.T. Sigler[16] and other investigators at Johns Hopkins University involved 216 families each with a Mongoloid child born and living in the city of Baltimore. The investigators reported that mothers of the Mongoloid children had been exposed to x-rays seven times as much as a group of control mothers. Furthermore, some studies[17] have shown an increase in the number of childhood malignancies including leukemia as a result of x-ray diagnostic exposure of the mother prior to conception.

There have been a number of publications recently which seem to confirm further a linear relationship between x-ray dose and effect all the way from the very high doses delivered to the survivors of the atomic bombings at Hiroshima and Nagasaki and for high doses delivered to certain tissues of the body during therapeutic treatment (such as that used for ankylosing spondylitis) to the low doses delivered in x-ray diagnosis. For example, R. Doll and P. G. Smith[18] report that in a series of 2,000 patients whose ovaries were irradiated with an estimated average of 136 rads (and only a very small dose to the bone marrow because of the small volume of tissue irradiated) to produce artificial menopause, there were six times as many deaths from leukemia and twice as many cancers of other types in the irradiated area as found in the control groups. They concluded that their observations are consistent with the hypothesis that the risk of leukemia is proportional to the gram-rad dose (i.e., the dose in rads multiplied by the grams of red marrow irradiated), irrespective of which volume of marrow is irradiated. Likewise, L. H. Hempelmann[19] published a paper that would tend to support a linear hypothesis for radiation-induced thyroid cancer over the wide range of 20 to 1,200 rads of external dose to the thyroid glands.

REDUCING THE RISK

The problem of assigning quantitative values to the benefits and risks and weighing one against the other as illustrated in Figure 1 is not an easy one. I believe that at present the scales in Figure 1 swing down heavily on the benefit side of the balance, and there is no doubt that the medical benefits far exceed the medical risks. I know, however, of no reliable data relative to the number of lives saved each year from the medical use of diagnostic x-rays. For lack of a known value, we might arbitrarily assume a number—for example, 100,000—of lives saved each year from the diagnostic use of x-rays. Regardless of what estimates are used or the arbitrariness of the number selected, it is evident that medical diagnosis is responsible for the saving of many thousands of lives each year. On the other hand, unnecessary diagnostic x-ray exposure to the population very probably accounts for the loss of thousands of lives each year. Just because the medical x-ray facilities in a city are responsible, for example, for saving ten or twenty lives each year, this in no way justifies the loss of one to five lives in this same period because of the use of poor equipment and improper techniques. The average diagnostic dose to the population could be reduced to less than 10 percent of its present value without any curtailment in the beneficial uses of diagnostic x-rays, while at the same time enhancing and immensely improving diagnostic x-rays. Techniques for reducing radiation exposure in medical and dental practice are summarized in Table 5.

There are other areas in which radiation exposure may be reduced. It has been encouraging during the past few years that a large number of colleges and universities throughout the world have established courses in health physics. There is considerable demand for health physicists not only to teach courses and conduct health physics research but also to serve as radiation protection officers to assure the safety of the students, faculty, and others who might be exposed to excessive radiation from university-owned and operated reactors, accelerators, x-ray machines, diffraction devices, isotope applications and all sorts of electronic equipment such as electron microscopes, voltage regulators, rectifiers,

BENEFITS	RISKS
Good Health—Entertainment— Employment—Modern Conveniences— Affluent Society	Sickness and Suffering—Deformities and Physical Handicaps—Life Shortening and Early Death
Medical X-Ray Treatment of diseases Medical diagnosis	
Color Television Educational programs News and political information Entertainment	
Nuclear Power Cheap electricity Reduction in air pollution	**Cancer** Leukemia Central nervous system cancer Bone Tumor Thyroid cancer Lung carcinoma
Industrial X-Ray Locate metallurgical flaws (prevent accidents)	
Microwave Ovens Safer and quicker preparation of food	**Eye Cataract**
Ultraviolet Radiation Destroy bacteria in operating rooms	**Life Shortening**
Radar Improved and safer air transportation	**Damage to Unborn Children** Mongoloidism Microcephaly (abnormal smallness of head) Various forms of cancer
Laser Improved communications	
Radioisotopes Medical diagnosis and treatment, power source for heart pump, etc.	**Genetic Mutations** Fetal and infant deaths Deformities (physical and mental)

Figure 1

vacuum condensers, vacuum switches, lasers, radar, and microwave ovens. One of the more serious health physics education problems is the fact that there are many industries, laboratories, universities, hospitals, etc., where health physics programs are needed urgently, but those in charge of the operations are not sufficiently aware of this need, or they are attempting to carry out health physics programs with untrained and improperly qualified personnel. This is particularly true of some of the nuclear power companies in the United States that would rather "retread" some of their older and less gainfully engaged employees than hire more competent and adequately trained health physicists.

TABLE 5

RADIATION EXPOSURE–SOME PROBLEMS AND SOLUTIONS

Typical Problems	Suggested Solution
1. Some x-ray equipment is being imported into the United States which does not contain meters to indicate x-ray current and voltage.	1. Prohibit import of such equipment.
2. Only the state of California now requires in medical schools education and training in x-rays and their safe use and state board examinations in these subjects.	2. Bring about such programs in remaining 49 states.
3. Only New York, New Jersey and California now require of x-ray technologists education, training and certification in x-rays and their safe use.	3. Bring about such programs in remaining 47 states.
4. Image intensifiers have made it possible to reduce dose to patient from fluoroscopic examinations by a factor of 100 or more. However, in many cases this factor is lost completely because some radiologists now fail to use equipment properly.	4. Gain this factor of 100 in patient dose reduction by properly directed educational programs (and, if necessary, inspection programs).
5. There is a shortage of radiologists and properly qualified x-ray technologists. These shortages would perhaps decrease by taking suggested measures 2, 3 and 4 above.	5. Intensify educational programs. Add the rank of senior x-ray technologist with a minimum of four years of special training. Permit these senior x-ray technologists to be completely responsible for care and operation of diagnostic x-ray equipment. This would upgrade the x-ray technologist profession and that of the radiologist. The radiologist could then concentrate on the more professional requirements of x-ray therapy, radiographic interpretation, etc.
6. Some medical institutions and doctors still require routine x-ray pelvic measurements in pregnancy cases.	6. Strongly discourage practice.
7. In many medical and dental radiograms, the cross-sectioned area of x-ray beam is two or more times the area of the film.	7. Require use of proper diaphragm, cones and collimators (including rectangular precision collimators and automatic collimators).

8. Fluoroscopic equipment improperly used, e.g. to fluoroscope music students to follow progress in proper use of throat muscles or to inspect employees leaving a factory to discourage stealing tools, etc.	8. Prohibit such use.

On some very crude assumptions, I have estimated that the nuclear power industry in the United States should have in its present employ approximately 400 health physicists; yet I estimate this number is only about 50. At this time when there is so much public concern about the possible risks from nuclear power plants, I know of no better investment the power companies could make than to strengthen their health physics organizations in order to develop a better understanding and appreciation of the problems and convince the public that radiation protection really is being taken seriously and provided for adequately by the power industry.

Likewise, radiation protection programs in many cities, states, and countries are falling far behind for lack of proper financing and well-trained health physicists. Many radiation-producing devices are surveyed and calibrated on a very infrequent basis, if at all. Mass chest x-ray programs are sometimes conducted where one might question the need, in spite of the fact the U.S. Public Health Service has indicated that mass chest x-ray programs should not be given to all population groups,[20] but only to those groups where the incidence of tuberculosis is high. Often, excessive use is made of chest x-ray surveys in spite of the fact that the World Health Organization[21] has pointed out that "attempts have been made to use mass radiography for detecting lung cancer at an early stage, but the results have been relatively poor and little if any improvement in the prognosis has been achieved." Often, techniques and examination can be carried out with doses as low as 10 to 20 millirads. Although some mass chest x-ray programs are essential, it seems to me that the health physicist should insist on better justification for programs where equipment and techniques arc used which deliver doses that are a factor of 10 to 100 times those delivered by better techniques and equipment. In some cases, toothpaste surveys have been conducted among thousands of children in which toothpaste is supplied free to the children in a city school system for a year, and then the children are subject to a series of dental x-rays ostensibly to determine which toothpaste results in a lesser number of caries. Since these studies usually are not scientific in nature and since the equipment employed in x-raying the teeth often has not been properly evaluated, calibrated and inspected before use, it is my opinion that this risk of x-ray damage to young children is unwarranted. It seems to me that frequently the primary purpose of such surveys may be to provide information for commercial TV and radio advertisements to increase the sales of particular brands of toothpaste. In my opinion, such programs should not be approved unless they have been carefully evaluated and appropriately justified. One institution,[22] North Texas State University, is using fluoroscopic x-ray equipment in the music department to observe the throats and jaws of the students to determine their progress in using various musical instruments. I would be strongly inclined to discourage such use of x-rays for many of the same reasons some of us had a part in discouraging the use of shoe-fitting x-ray machines a couple of decades ago.

TV EXPOSURE

Radiation hazards of color television have probably received more publicity than is warranted; in the vast majority of cases exposures from these sets are extremely low. Although H. J. L. Rechen and his colleagues[23] have shown that the voltage regulator tube in some makes of color television sets can be selected and adjusted in such a manner as to give a dose as high as 800,000 millirads per hour at the bottom of the receiver, I doubt that there have been very much, if any, color television sets approaching this condition. The dose delivered by most color television sets is almost negligible. A survey of the U.S. Public Health Service in the metropolitan area of Washington, D.C.,[24] for example, indicated that only about 6 percent of these sets exceeded the maximum permissible level set by the National Council on Radiation Protection of 0.5 millirad per hour at five centimeters (about two inches) from any accessible point on the surface of the receiver, and only two out of 1,124 sets inspected exceeded 12.5 millirads per hour (the full-scale reading of the survey instrument used). However, in my opinion, even this low exposure is totally unwarranted, because it represents unnecessary exposure and a potential for radiation damage to many millions of children who sit for hours each day only a few feet from the screens of the twenty million color TV sets in the United States.

During the past few years, there has been rapid expansion in the types and number of energy sources which produce exposure to ionizing radiation. Many of these are not commonly recognized or clearly identified as potential sources of serious radiation exposure. For example, the high-voltage vacuum switch is commonly used in various countries of the world as a convenient means of breaking the high potential side of an electrical circuit. These devices are used in industries, hospitals, and universities. J.A. Auxier and his colleagues[25] have tested a number of these and have found some delivering absorbed doses as high as one rad per hour at ten feet. This terrific dose rate (about two million times the permissible nonoccupational rate at one foot from the switch) is delivered in the vicinity of these and other similar electronic products in spite of the fact that the specifications and other literature furnished by the vendor mention nothing about the fact that these devices can emit x-rays.

It is even conceivable that after a thorough evaluation of the problem has been made, consideration will be given to reducing the natural background radiation dose to the population by recommending that certain building materials that are high in uranium and thorium ores be avoided as construction material for homes, schools, and factories. Such precautionary measures could be significant; for example, in Tennessee, cement blocks are often made from Conasauga shale, and in Florida these blocks are sometimes made from phosphate rock. Both of these minerals contain a fairly high concentration of uranium ores, and in homes having a recirculating air supply, the radon gas from the uranium seeps out of these blocks and reaches equilibrium with its daughter products which are continuously recycled in the atmosphere. It has been shown[26] that in such homes the lung dose is frequently ten times the average dose.

From the above discussion, I believe it is evident that efforts should be made to avoid even very low levels of unnecessary radiation exposure to large numbers of the population. It must be kept in mind, however, that ionizing radiation is just one of many risks in modern society, and we must not attempt to reduce to zero the risks from any one potential source of injury at the expense of seriously increasing other risks. In considering the radioactive contamination we will allow in a river system or the dose that will be permitted to a critical segment of the population from nuclear power production, for instance, we must consider, also, the risks from sulfur dioxide and oxides of nitrogen in the environment and increasing the cost of electricity. All these risks must be related in an effort to maximize the overall benefits to all members of the population.

NOTES

1. Morgan, K.A., "Ionizing Radiation: Benefits Versus Risks," *Health Physics Journal,* 17 (4) :539, 1969.
2. Gitlin, J.N., and P.S. Lawrence, *Population Exposure to X-Rays, U.S. 1964,* Public Health Service Publication No. 1519, U.S. Government Printing Office, Washington, D.C. Baltz, Hanson, "Common Causes of Excessive Patient Exposure in Diagnostic Radiology," *New England Journal of Medicine,* 271:1184, December 3, 1964.
3. Gitlin and Lawrence, *loc cit.*
4. Medwedeff, F.M. and P.D. Elcan, "A Precision Technic to Minimize Radiation," *Dental Survey,* October 1967.
5. National Advisory Committee on Radiation, R.H. Morgan, chairman, U.S. Department of Health, Education & Welfare, *Protecting and Improving Health Through the Radiological Services,* April 1966.

6. Committee of the International Commission on Radiological Protection, R.H. Mole, chairman, *Radiosensitivity and Spatial Distribution of Dose*, ICRP Publication 14, Pergamon Press, London, 1969, p. 40.

7. *Recommendations of the International Commission on Radiological Protection*, ICRP Publication 9, Pergamon Press, London, 1966.

8. *Recommendations of the International Commission on Radiological Protection*, ICRP Publication 1, Pergamon Press, London, 1959.

9. Morgan, K.Z., "Reduction of Unnecessary Medical Exposures," testimony before the Senate Commerce Committee on Senate Bill S.2067, August 28, 1967. Morgan, K.Z., "Population Exposure to Diagnostic X-Rays and the Resultant Damage Can be Reduced to 10% of Their Present Levels While at the Same Time Increasing the Quality and Amount of Diagnostic Information," testimony before the House of Representatives on H.R. 10790, October 11, 1967.

10. Adrian, G.M., "Hazards and Dose to the Whole Population from Ionizing Radiations," *Annals of Occupational Hygiene, 9:83, 1966.*

11. *Population Dose from X-Rays, U.S., 1964*, U.S. Public Health Service Publication No. 2001, October 1969.

12. *Report of the United Nations Scientific Committee on the Effects of Atomic Radiation*, Supplement 17, A/3838, 1958; Supplement 16, A/5216, 1962; Supplement 14, A/5814, 1964; Supplement 14, A/6314, 1966, United Nations, New York.

13. Russell, W.L., "Studies in Mammalian Radiation Genetics," *Nucleonics*, 23(1) :53, 1965.

14. Division of Biology and Medicine, *Prenatal X-Ray and Childhood Neoplasia*, U.S. Atomic Energy Commission Report, TID-12373, April 1, 1961.

15. MacMahan, Brian, "X-Ray Exposure and Malignancy," *Journal of the American Medical Association*, 183:721, 1963.

16. Sigler, A.T., *Public Health Reports*, 81:225, March 1966.

17. Stewart, A. et al., "A Survey of Childhood Malignancies," *British Medical Journal*, p. 1495, 1958. Graham, S. et al., "Preconception, Intrauterine, and Postnatal Irradiation as Related to Leukemia," *Epidemiological Approaches to the Study of Cancer and Other Chronic Diseases*, NCI Monograph 19, January 1966.

18. Doll, R. and P.G. Smith, "The Long-Term Effects of X Irradiation in Patients Treated for Metropathia Haemorrhagica," *British Journal of Radiology*, 41:362, May 1968.

19. Hempelmann, L.H., "Risk of Thyroid Neoplasms After Irradiation in Childhood," *Science*, 160:159, April 12, 1968.

20. Chadwick, D.R., "Highlights of the U.S. Public Health Service X-Ray Exposure Study," presented at the 29th Annual Meeting of the Canadian Association of Radiologists, Montreal, Canada, March 5, 1966.

21. "The Early Detection of Cancer," *WHO Chronicle*, 23 (12) :537, 1969.

22. "Transparent Man with a Horn," *The North Texan*, 19 (5) :7, North Texas State University, Denton, October 1968.

23. Rechen, H.J.L. et al., "Measurements of X-Ray Exposure from a Home Color Television Receiver," *Radiological Health Data and Reports*, p. 687, December 1967.

24. U.S. Health Service, *A Survey of X-Radiation from Color Television Sets in the Washington, D.C., Metropolitan Area*, Rockville, Maryland, March 1968.

25. Auxier, J.A. and F.F. Haywood, unpublished data, Health Physics Division, Oak Ridge National Laboratory, Oak Ridge, Tennessee, 1968.
26. Gabrysh, A.F. and F.J. Davis, "Radon Released from Concrete in Radiant Heating," *Nucleonics,* p. 50, January 1955. Gabrysh, A.F. and F.J. Davis, "Radiation Exposure from Radiant Heating," *Civil Engineering,* 89:839, December 1954, Hultqvist, B., "Studies on Naturally Occurring Ionizing Radiations," *Almqvist & Wiksells Boktryckeri Ab, 1956.*
27. *Population Dose from X-Rays, U.S., 1964,* U.S. Public Health Service Publication No. 2001, October 1969.
28. Estimate by K.Z. Morgan from Gitlin and Lawrence, *loc. cit.* and Laughlin and Pullman Report NAS-NRC, March 1957.
29. Estimate by Karl Z. Morgan from *Report of the United Nations Scientific Committee on the Effects of Atomic Radiation, loc. cit.* Adrian Report, "Radiological Hazards to Patients," 1966. Gitlin and Lawrence, *loc. cit.*
30. Value of mrem/yr for weapons fallout radiation was calculated by W.D. Cottrell of the ORNL Health Physics Division. Actually, the calculations indicated the gonad and total body dose from ^{137}Cs to be 1.2 mrem in 1966, 0.68 mrem in 1967 and 0.54 mrem in 1968. The average bone dose was calculated to be 3.6 mrem in 1966, 2.8 mrem in 1967 and 2.3 mrem in 1968.
31. Estimate by K.Z. Morgan from a number of reports.
32. *Report of the United Nations Scientific Committee on the Effects of Atomic Radiation,* Supplement 16, *loc. cit.*
33. Value from U.S. Public Health Service preliminary reports.
34. Estimate by K.Z. Morgan from *Report of the United Nations Scientific Committee on the Effects of Atomic Radiation,* Supplement 16, *loc. cit.* and from the Adrian Report, *loc. cit.*
35. Morgan, K.Z., and J.E. Turner, eds., *Principles of Radiation Protection,* John Wiley and Sons, Inc., New York, 1967.

V. UNDERSTANDING TOXIC

SUBSTANCE POLLUTION

Toxic Substances: Chemicals and Metals

Toxic Substances Are Entering The Environment

About 2 million chemical compounds are known, and several thousand new chemicals are discovered each year. Most new compounds are laboratory curiosities that will never be produced commercially. However, several hundred of these new chemicals are introduced into commercial use annually. Of particular concern because of their rapidly increasing number and use are the metals, metallic compounds, and synthetic organic compounds.

U.S. consumption of metals with known toxic effects has increased greatly in the last 20 years. The data on use underestimate the increasing pervasiveness of metals in our environment because many new metallic compounds are being formulated and used in an ever widening variety of new products.

Similarly, use of synthetic organic chemicals is growing rapidly. Over 9,000 synthetic compounds are now in commercial use in amounts of over 1,000 pounds each per year. In 1968, they totaled nearly 120 billion pounds—a 15 percent increase over 1967 and a 161 percent increase over 10 years ago.

Although many of these substances are not toxic, the sheer number of them, their increasing diversity and use, and the environmental problems already encountered from some indicate the existence of a problem.

These substances enter man's environment—and man himself—through complex and interrelated pathways. Present in air, water, soil, consumer products, and food, they pervade our environment. They often become concentrated through the food chain—with minute quantities being magnified thousands of times as they are consumed by higher forms of life. Increasingly, all forms of life are being exposed to potentially toxic substances.

These Substances Can Have Severe Effects

The environmental effects of most of the substances discussed . . . are not well understood. Testing has largely been confined to their acute effects, and knowledge of the chronic, long-term effects, such as genetic mutation, is

Excerpts from: *Toxic Substances,* Council on Environmental Quality, April 1971.

inadequate. Although far from complete, available data indicate the potential or actual danger of a number of these substances.

Many serious effects, including those resulting in cancer (carcinogenicity), genetic mutations which cause permanent and transmissible change in the genes of offspring from those of the parent (mutagenicity), and production of physical or biochemical defects in an offspring (teratogenicity) can occur from metals, their compounds, and synthetic organic compounds. In general, we do not know which chemicals cause such effects or the levels that a given chemical must reach before the effects occur.

The problem is complicated by the chemical changes which may occur once toxic substances enter the environment. They can become more toxic through modification in the ecosystem or as a result of synergistic actions with other substances.

Wildlife and fish populations are also being exposed to these substances, and some species have already been severely damaged by such exposure.

Recent incidents of mercury and other contamination of the environment and the diversity and quantities of toxic and potentially toxic substances entering the environment indicate the extent of this growing national problem. Action is needed to prevent damage to man's health and the environment. New regulatory authority, improved research, and better monitoring systems have been recommended and must be implemented now if protection is to be provided.

The approach called for in the Toxic Substances Control Act is a new way of looking at environmental problems. Rather than dealing with pollutants as they appear in air, in water, and on land, it represents a systematic and comprehensive approach to the problem. It relies on understanding the flow of potentially toxic substances throughout the entire range of activity—from extraction to production to consumer use and to disposal. Only through such a comprehensive approach can we provide protection to man and his environment. In the last few years, we have identified the enormity of the problem; we have developed the institutional capability through the creation of EPA to look comprehensively at pollution of the environment. The time has come for an action program to control the use of toxic substances.

Interactions Within The Environment

After substances enter the environment, they may be diluted or concentrated by physical forces, and they may undergo chemical changes, including combination with other chemicals, that affect their toxicity. The substances may be picked up by living organisms which may further change and either store or eliminate them.

The results of the interaction between living organisms and chemical substances are often unpredictable, but such interaction may produce materials that are more dangerous than the initial pollutants. One example is inorganic mercury, which was thought to settle safely into the bottom sediments when discharged into water. Anaerobic bacteria are now known to convert inorganic mercury into very toxic and soluble organic mercury compounds, such as methylmercury, which pass through the food chain by aquatic algae and by fish, eventually reaching man.

DDT, another example, is nearly insoluble in water. It occurs in high concentrations among some fish-eating birds as a result of two factors: DDT's solubility in fats is much higher than in water, and plankton, shellfish, and fish generally pass successively higher concentrations of DDT on to the organism next in the food chain. Polychlorinated biphenyls (PCB's), which are chemically similar to DDT, have been found in similar association with marine food chains. Oysters exposed to one type of PCB for 96 hours accumulated the substance to a level 3,300 times that of the ambient water.

Synergism is another complicating interaction. Two or more compounds acting together may have an effect on organisms greater than the sum of their separate effects. For example, the toxic effects of mercuric salts are accentuated by the presence of trace amounts of copper. Cadmium acts as a synergist with zinc and cyanide in the aquatic environment to increase toxicity. Conversely, sometimes the presence of one substance lessens the effect of another substance on an organism. Arsenic, a toxic substance itself, counteracts the toxicity of selenium and has been added to poultry and cattle feed in areas where animal feeds are naturally high in selenium.

EFFECTS OF TOXIC SUBSTANCES

As noted earlier, metals, unlike synthetic organic compounds, have always been present in the environment, and living organisms—including man—have evolved in their presence. Blood and body tissues are composed of a complex mixture of elemental substances, including the metals. Some metals are essential to life at low concentrations but are toxic at higher concentrations. Further, the form in which the metal occurs—as a pure metal, an inorganic metallic compound, or an organic metallic compound—strongly influences its toxicity. Thus the danger of metals to man depends on their concentration and chemical form.

Most synthetic organic substances are not essential to life, though many share with metals the characteristic of toxicity. As with metals, the concentration and type of exposure to a particular synthetic organic substance are key factors in determining its effects.

The total effect of all toxic substances on a single species, say, man, is impossible to quantify with accuracy because of our lack of knowledge about the effects of toxic substances. Although many substances in the environment can cause death or injury if man is exposed to them in sufficiently high concentrations, the effects of long-term exposure to low levels of such substances, singly or in combination, are generally unknown. A standard text on the dangers of commercial products rates the toxicity of more than 1,000 commercially used chemical compounds, most of which are toxic to man at high levels of exposure. However, the long-term effects of low levels are known for only a few.

Although lack of effort partially accounts for this paucity of knowledge, our ignorance also stems from the many difficulties inherent in testing for adverse effects. The large number of chemicals that should be evaluated by long-term laboratory experiments requiring many test animals is a serious limiting factor. Extrapolation of data on dose effects obtained from animal studies to man must consider many species variations in response to exposure from toxic substances. Substances rarely occur in the environment in isolation, so that possible synergism or antagonism of two or more substances adds to the difficulty of adequate testing and of interpretation of field results.

Difficult choices must also be made in determining the effects or biological end points to be examined. Biological end points are often determined from such irreversible effects as carcinogenesis, mutagenesis, and teratogenesis.

Carcinogenesis is the ability of a substance to cause cancer. Chemical mutagenesis is the induction in protoplasm of genetic mutations by a substance. These can be permanent and transmissible changes in the genes of an offspring from those of the parents of earlier generations. Teratogenesis is the production of physical or biochemical defects in an offspring during gestation; it is limited to a particular child. During the last decade, there were many deformed infants born of women who had ingested the drug thalidomide during pregnancy—a vivid example of teratogenesis.

The effects of any given substance may vary among individuals and among species. Differences in effects are a function of age, sex, health condition and history, stress, different metabolic patterns in different species, and other less understood factors. Further, we often do not know how to apply to humans the results from experiments with laboratory animals. If a substance produces cancer in mice, will it produce human cancers? How do we extrapolate the level of a substance required to produce a given effect in mice to the level that will produce the same effect in man? If mice are not affected by a substance, is that substance also safe for humans?

All these difficulties contribute to the dearth of knowledge concerning the biological effects of many environmental contaminants and particularly the toxic substances discussed in this report. But we do understand enough to know that many substances may significantly threaten man and the environment.

Many useful data on health effects of toxic substances derive from studies of occupational exposure. Commonly, the levels of exposure are much higher at the workplace than in the total environment, and the data gathered on exposed groups of workers can contribute to understanding effects on the general population. However, even here caution must be exercised in interpreting the results for nonindustrial groups who are exposed to lower concentrations and whose level of health may not match that of the industrial worker.

Food

INTRODUCTION

A basic need of man is safe, wholesome, nutritious food. However, food can be a source of disease agents, toxins, poisons, and malnutrition. Authorities estimate that two to ten million people in this country contract some form of food-borne disease annually. The economic loss as a result of this, in terms of drain on our personal health care resources and loss in productive effort, amounts to billions of dollars each year. Development of new foods and widespread use of new technology in the food industry contribute to a proliferation of products whose health impact is relatively unknown. Filthy or decomposed raw materials or existence of insanitary conditions in food manufacture and processing plants are conditions no longer acceptable to the consumer.

Rapidly advancing nutritional knowledge has brought about improvement in the quality of our diet, leading to a remarkable decrease of nutritional deficiency diseases. For example, pellagra, which once claimed more than 7,000 lives yearly, is now so rare that it is not even catalogued in the current National Nutritional Survey. Improvement must be maintained and extended by ensuring that nutrients are not destroyed by preparation, processing, storage, or product deterioration. Manufacturers who introduce new foods or new food processing techniques should be provided guidelines for nutritional quality which must be provided by each such food.

Food protection has become sufficiently complex to defy complete control at any one level of government. Sanitation problems can occur in any of 45,000 food processing establishments, or among 25,000 manufacturers, warehouses, and other types of firms. In addition, there are approximately 500,000 food service establishments in the United States in which contamination may occur. There is a need to develop, conduct, coordinate and strengthen programs to provide more comprehensive protection throughout the food chain from

Excerpts from *Environmental Health Planning,* U.S. Department of Health, Education and Welfare, Public Health Service Publication 2120, Bureau of Community Environmental Management, 1971.

production through consumption. Environmental health agencies have a responsibility to see that this protection is provided, either directly or through other competent agencies..

Mission

The primary elements which comprise the mission of food protection are:

1. To assure wholesome and clean food free from unsafe bacterial and chemical contamination, filth, and natural or added deleterious substances.
2. To assure adequate nutrition by ensuring compliance of foods with established nutritional quality guidelines, and with standards of quality and identity, and by ensuring that foods marketed for special purposes are suitably labeled to fully inform as to their nutritional attributes.
3. To prevent food-borne disease transmission and prevent significant microbiological and chemical contamination and decomposition during production, processing, distribution, storage, preparation, and service.

PROBLEMS

The following are the primary problems of concern to state and local food regulatory agencies:

1. *Microbiological Contamination.* It is estimated that up to ten million Americans suffer from food-borne illness annually. Salmonellosis, shigellosis, illness due to *Clostridium perfringens, Vibrio* and viruses, and food poisonings caused by *Staphylococcus* and *Clostridium botulinus* toxins are transmitted through contaminated foods. Development of new foods, changing distribution and delivery systems, centralizations of food processing, and widespread use of new technologies and procedures result in increased potential for food-borne illness. Problems of food sanitation are complicated by the use of filthy or decomposed raw materials or by insanitary conditions in food manufacture, processing, and delivery systems which permit finished product contamination. This contamination often has detrimental health implications. Thus, sanitation is an integral part of all other food programs.
2. *Chemical Additives Contamination.* The average American is said to consume three pounds of chemical additives in his food each year. Food protection demands assurance that the additive performs its intended use, and that maximum level of each additive introduced into the total food does not exceed established tolerance. Only approved additives are to be used. Ingestion of naturally occurring toxins such as aflatoxin, fish and shellfish toxins, and plant poisons, is a significant problem. Certain essential nutrients may be used in excessive and potentially toxic amounts because

of ignorance, individual taste or well-meaning zeal. These include salt, various amino acids for flavor or technological use, vitamins and mineral essentials. (For discussion of pesticides in food refer to chapter on "Pesticides.")

3. *Nutritional Adequacy and Availability.* "Nutritional quackery," (deceptive and misleading claims) is a major problem and costs American consumers as much as $500 million a year. This figure does not include slack fill, substitution of cheaper ingredients, or low drained weights which represent economic frauds. Adequate food standards protect the health as well as the pocketbook of consumers, who otherwise might fail to obtain expected nutrients. If the diet is marginal or submarginal, this could have serious health implications.

Another problem is protection of nutrients from loss due to improper storage, excessive shelf life, rancidity, or new processes. Close cooperation is needed with state agriculture and extension services as well as food science and food technology and home economics departments in universities and colleges. Individuals responsible for food preparation and handling in public eating establishments must be made aware of the importance of protecting foods from nutritional deterioration through poor handling during preparation. This problem has not yet been adequately explained to the food industry and food handling detrimental to preservation of nutritional quality is still common in food service establishments.

Food Toxicology: Safety of Food Additives

J. M. Coon

The current wave of public anxiety relating to chemical additives and pesticide residues in foods is an unfortunate phenomenon. It has been generated primarily from the publicity arising from recent experimental findings relating to the potential hazards of several specific chemical substances associated with our foods, notably DDT, the cyclamates, and monosodium glutamate. The recent official bans or restrictions of the use of DDT and cyclamates have brought the controversy to a boil, resulting in a spillover of concern for food additives and pesticides in our food supply. The development of such a furor is indeed surprising in view of the lack of evidence that the presence of any of these agents in foods over many years has been responsible for any adverse effects in the human consumer.

But since the issues involved pertain to the health of the general consumer, it behooves the physician to be able to give sound advice to his questioning and worried patients on the basis of fact and established toxicologic principles. After all, the misinformation and misinterpretations in this area that have become a substantial part of the patient's daily reading diet may be hazardous to his health. In this case, the indicated treatment becomes a matter of reassuring the patient that qualified scientists, government officials, and the food industry are concerned, active, and effective in preventing dangerous amounts of chemicals from entering his food supply.

Food additives and pesticide residues should be viewed in the context of the chemical makeup of the specific foods in which they are present and of the total diet. All foods in their natural state are complex mixtures of chemical substances, only a relatively small number of which are the nutrient components. By far the largest number are nonnutrient substances that provide desirable color, flavor, odor, form, or consistency or are of no known functional value whatever. Many of the nutrient, as well as the known nonnutrient, components of natural food products have recognized toxic properties, and many others that have not been identified chemically are completely unknown toxicologically. It is fair to say that the chemicals naturally present in foods

Reprinted by permission from *Modern Medicine,* November 30, 1970, pp. 103-108.

constitute a much greater toxicologic unknown than do chemicals used by man to improve his food supply. Natural products that are now widely used as foods have been accepted as safe, not on the basis of scientific tests but on the basis of long experience throughout history that has taught man what may be consumed in reasonable amounts without causing injury. On the other hand, the food additives that man puts into, or the pesticides that he allows to enter, foods are scientifically evaluated for safety for their intended uses, and the amounts permitted in any food are in most cases miniscule when compared in perspective with the natural composition of a given food or of the total diet.

This does not mean that we need not watch carefully what enters foods as a result of man's food production and processing activities. The presence of many toxic components in natural food products should be considered a logical reason for avoiding the addition of harmful amounts of other substances. We must have stringent laws to control these activities. Fortunately, we do have such laws, which appear to have been effective and are for the most part reasonable. But there are recognized gaps in our knowledge of the subtle effects of chemicals in the body, how to interpret observed effects in the interest of human health, and how to devise tests that will provide data that can be used with maximum confidence in the assessment of safety. For these reasons, continued research is necessary to establish the soundest possible basis for confidence in the safety of our food supply.

For our present purpose, we may define a food additive, in its broadest sense, as any substance that, as used by man, enters food in any of the various stages of its production, processing, packaging, or storing and remains in the food at the time of consumption. Under this definition a substance may be referred to as a *direct* or an *indirect* food additive.

The direct additives are deliberately used in food processing to enhance or conserve the nutritional value or to improve or maintain the desirable chemical and physical characteristics of the food, such as flavor, color, texture, and consistency. These agents or their derivatives are intended to remain in the foods at the time of consumption.

The indirect additives enter and remain in foods as a result of their use as pesticides or fertilizers, after their addition to animal feeds, from synthetic or chemically processed packaging materials, or through chemical changes wrought in foods by processing methods, including preservation by ionizing radiation. Such substances are essentially contaminants and have no function in the final food product.

Most of the present controversy that rages over chemicals in foods involves the direct food additives. It is estimated that approximately 2,000 different materials are used by the industry to enhance the quality, facilitate the processing, and increase the consumer acceptability of foods. A wide variety of functions is performed by these agents. They may be nutrients or dietary supplements, flavors, acidifiers, alkalizers, buffers, sweeteners, stabilizers, thickeners, emulsifiers, preservatives, antioxidants, or antimicrobial agents. Or they may be used for their anticaking, texturizing, bleaching, coloring or color fixative, maturing, curing, leavening, humectant, solvent, or sequestrant properties.

More than half of these substances are employed for flavoring purposes alone, and many of these are natural products or their extracts, things that have been used for generations, such as anise, bay, and clove and down through a long list to thyme, vanilla, and zedoary bark. Many specific chemicals—organic acids, alcohols, esters, aldehydes, ketones, phenols, terpenes, sulfur compounds, essential oils, resin, oleresins, etc.—are also used after synthesis or separation from their natural sources, having been identified as responsible for the gustatory properties of natural spices and seasonings or of natural food products. In fact, practically all of the more than 1,000 direct food additives used for flavoring purposes are natural products or chemicals identical to the components of natural products that have been used as, or in, foods for hundreds of years. Cyclamate and saccharin are notable exceptions, being synthetic substances not occurring naturally.

To maintain a balanced view of flavoring agents as a class of food additives, it should be stated that any one specific product or chemical entity can readily be demonstrated to have toxic properties if fed to experimental animals in large enough amounts. No hazard has been associated with their reasonable use in the human diet, however, because the discrete chemicals involved achieve their flavoring functions in extremely minute and toxicologically insignificant amounts. Again, cyclamate and saccharin might be considered exceptions, though no proof has been established that these are hazardous to man under the conditions of their past or present use.

The second largest class of food additives are the nutrients and dietary supplements, such as numerous preparations of vitamins, minerals, and other essential elements and their simple inorganic compounds and amino acids. Comprising the other categories of additives are many simple inorganic and organic acids and their salts, esters of fatty acids, proteins, carbohydrates, polysaccharides, and natural coloring materials. In viewing these lists of substances, one sees that most of them are compounds or derivatives of compounds that either are essential for good nutrition, are natural constituents of the human body, or have been present in the human diet through the ages. A surprisingly few direct food additives are synthetic chemicals that are not present in our natural environment.

It should be emphasized that long-continued and widespread dietary use of a substance without evidence of adverse effects does not by itself constitute proof of its safety, whether its source be natural or synthetic. For example, we do not yet have adequate scientific proof of the safety of saccharin, though it has been used extensively in many countries for eighty years with no sign of injury to the consumer becoming apparent. Long-delayed effects are frequently difficult to relate to their specific causes. Thus, it is conceivable that injuries due to unrecognized causes have been produced by common materials that have long been considered safe as foods or for use in foods. In this regard we are concerned with cancer, genetic damage and birth defects, premature old age, cardiovascular, endocrine, and mental disorders, and other human ills of unexplained etiology.

In spite of these considerations, there is no good reason to believe that the general health of the population has declined, as some would claim, as a result of the presence of the direct and indirect food additives in its diet or to doubt that our dietary as a whole is as safe and wholesome as it has ever been, if not more so. Certainly, more is being done now than ever before to achieve the latter.

If the public were made more aware of the scientific activities and governmental controls directed toward the safety of its food supply, it would know that its health in this respect is being looked after with much vigor. Three amendments to the Federal Food, Drug, and Cosmetic Act of 1938 control the uses of additives in food processing and of chemicals as pesticides in food production. These are the Pesticide Amendment of 1954, the Food Additive Amendment of 1958, and the Color Additive Amendment of 1960. These laws require from the producer appropriate evidence that any substance it wishes to use will be safe for the uses for which it is proposed. If the Food and Drug Administration approves the substance, it then issues regulations specifying the conditions of use, the particular foods in which it may be present, and the amount permitted. The controversial Delaney Clause of the Food Additive Amendment denies the use, in any amount, of any direct food additive that has been found to produce cancer in any species of test animal when fed at any level in its diet. In regard to pesticides also, official policy is to refuse permission for the use of any such agent that is carcinogenic in any test animal, at any dietary level, if detectable residues remain in the marketed foods from the crops to which it has been applied. This regulatory concept of no allowable presence of direct or indirect food additives is arbitrarily applied, even when scientific evidence and knowledge indicate that a hazard to man is highly unlikely under the proposed conditions of use of the substance in question.

The protocols for the evaluation of the safety of food additives and pesticides have become progressively more rigorous since the enactment of the Food Additive Amendment twelve years ago. For any new substance, extensive toxicological tests are required on at least two and preferably three species of animals. These include acute, short-term, and lifetime feeding studies; observations on growth, general well-being, and life-span; detailed histopathological examination of organs, tissues, and blood; organ function tests; exploration of possible effects on all aspects of reproductive physiology; tests for embryotoxicity, teratogenicity, and mutagenicity; studies on the patterns of absorption, distribution, metabolic fate, and excretion; a search for effects on various enzyme systems; and an investigation of potential toxicologic interactions with selected food chemicals and drugs. It is further recommended that small doses of the substance be tested in man for the way in which he handles it metabolically. If man is similar in this respect to one or more of the experimental animals studied, then the animal toxicity data can be more reliably extrapolated to man.

The essential purpose of the laboratory studies is to find the highest dietary level of the test substance that has no detectable adverse effect throughout the lifetime of the animal. This level, in the most sensitive of the species tested, is divided by 100 to arrive at what is considered the "safe" level in the human diet. The maximum allowable amounts (tolerances) in the specific foods in which the material is to be present are then set so that the "safe" level will not be exceeded in the diet of man. Frequently, if not usually, the amounts actually present in foods are substantially lower than those needed to achieve a "safe" level in the diet, because such amounts of the substance are not needed to accomplish the purpose for which its use is intended. From the results of recent surveys of pesticide residues in foods on the market, it has been estimated that the maximum daily intakes of all pesticides are well below their "safe" levels.

The interest of the consumer in the quality and safety of his food supply is abundantly served by a great array of scientific talent, time, energy, and financial resources. Besides the expert personnel of the Food and Drug Administration itself, committees of scientists of the National Academy of Sciences, the American Medical Association, and the Food and Agriculture Organization and World Health Organization of the United Nations, as well as many similar groups in other countries, continually review data pertaining to food safety. The information that such groups evaluate and interpret emanates from a multitude of laboratories distributed nationwide and worldwide in medical, veterinary, public health, and agricultural schools; in government agencies; and in independent and industrial research laboratories.

The Food Protection Committee of the Food and Nutrition Board of the National Academy of Sciences has worked since 1950 in an advisory capacity for government and industry in matters pertaining to food safety. One of its outstanding contributions is the *Food Chemicals Codex,* a compendium of food additives that provides chemical manufacturers and food processors with standards of identity and purity for food-grade chemicals similar to those available for drugs in the United States Pharmacopeia and National Formulary.

It seems amply evident that the relatively small component of man's chemical environment that is present in his food as a result of his use of additives and pesticides is more effectively studied, regulated, and controlled than any of the other aspects of that environment. In this area laws have been passed and actions taken *before* any damage was done to human health. If air and water pollution, the microbiological and natural hazards of foods, and other natural chemical hazards were as well controlled as food additives and pesticide residues in relation to human health, our causes for concern about our environment would virtually disappear.

The great number and variety of food additives and pesticides in use today is, in itself, the basis for much public alarm. The number is indeed impressive. But the very multiplicity of these agents provides a measure of protection according to the concept of the *safety in numbers*. Disregard for this concept led to the recent difficulties with the cyclamates and DDT. Without adequate competition from other agents, these materials became too widely used in excessive quantities. A recent report of the Joint FAO/WHO Expert Committee on Food Additives states: " ... an increase in the number of food additives on a permitted list does not imply an over-all increase in [the amount of] additives used; the different additives are largely used as alternatives ... From the toxicological point of view there is less likelihood of long exposure, or of high or cumulative dose levels being attained, if a wide range of substances is available for use. Similar considerations apply to pesticide residues." This principle is based on the fact that, though the human organism has a limited resistance against any given chemical substance, it can readily tolerate small amounts of many different ones taken simultaneously. The concurrent subliminal actions of small doses of many different toxic substances are not additive. If they were, we could not long endure even a well-balanced diet of natural food products completely free of man's additives and pesticides.

Another factor that serves to attenuate the force of the chemical attack upon the human organism in its environment is the frequency of occurrence of antagonistic interactions among chemicals present simultaneously in the body. This phenomenon is common and well known in the field of drugs, and there are many drugs that offset the actions of others. Similarly, DDT and most of the other so-called hard or persistent pesticides have been shown to promote the production of enzymes in the body that detoxify many other chemicals, including several of another important class of insecticides, the organophosphates such as parathion. Many examples of this balancing influence between foreign chemicals in the body could be cited. Our knowledge in this regard gives us good reason to believe there is more interference (antagonism) than there is collusion or reinforcement (synergism or potentiation) in the actions of the myriads of chemicals to which man is exposed.

It is a common impression that there is some insidious hazard associated with the consumption of a chemical that has been synthesized in the chemist's laboratory, even though it may be identical to a compound derived from natural sources. It is a toxicologic axiom, however, that any given chemical substance has exactly the same biological actions whether it is synthesized or isolated from its natural source. In regard to synthetic chemicals not known to occur in nature, such as a few of the food additives and many of the pesticides and drugs in use today, there is no evidence that the biochemical detoxication and other defense mechanisms of the body are generally less efficient in handling them than in handling the natural chemical components of our normal diet. Considering the tremendous number and variety of such substances in natural food products, many known and many more unknown, it is unlikely that man has synthesized chemicals that confront his physiological mechanisms with completely new and baffling detoxication problems.

The stringent laws and testing methods, the considerable scientific attention, the view in perspective of additives and pesticide residues in relation to our total chemical environment, and the various basic toxicologic principles as outlined above should provide adequate assurance of the safety of our food supply. Though there is pertinent knowledge that we lack and complacency is out of order, it is significant that no evidence has yet come to light that the public health is adversely affected by the unnatural chemicals in the food supply and that no outbreaks of injury have been related to the proper use of these materials. We do not have *absolute* proof of the *absolute* safety of any given substance in use, as some have demanded we must have, but absolutism in this respect is impossible—a will-o'-the-wisp. The application of the rules of reason and common sense, based on the scientific knowledge we now have plus what we hope to gain, should insure the maintenance of our good record of food safety.

The advantages achieved by the use of food additives and pesticides far outweigh any known risks. They have improved the quality, increased the quantity, availability, and acceptability, and kept down the cost of the basic elements of the food supply. The health risks of poor eating habits certainly far exceed those involved in the presence of food additives and pesticide residues in our daily diet.

Pesticides

INTRODUCTION

Today man is exposed to an ever increasing number and variety of chemicals, one group of which is pesticides.[1] Although pesticide chemicals were known and used before World War II, their use has increased significantly. New, more toxic compounds, such as the synthetic organic pesticides have largely replaced the older compounds. Little information is available to evaluate the hazards associated with use of the newer products. Our society has gained tremendous benefits from the use of pesticides, fungicides, herbicides and plant growth regulators to prevent vector-borne disease, to control insect pests, and to increase quantity and quality of foods and fibers. The need to use pesticides and other pest-control chemicals will continue to increase for the foreseeable future. However, recent evidence indicates a need to be concerned about unintentional effects of pesticides on human health and on various life forms within the environment. Residues have been found in human and other animal tissues, in food, clothing, water, soil, and air. It is apparent that the benefits of using pesticides must be considered in the context of the present and potential risks of pesticide usage. Corrective action must be taken now to protect the health of man and prevent further environmental pollution from pesticide residues.

Mission

The mission of a pesticide control program is to protect man and his environment from the adverse effects of pesticides. National pesticide control efforts include:

1. Determining pesticide use patterns most advantageous to man and his environment.

Excerpts from *Environmental Health Planning,* U.S. Department of Health, Education and Welfare, Public Health Service Publication 2120, Bureau of Community Environmental Management, 1971.

[1]The term "pesticide" means such substances as insecticides, fungicides, rodenticides, herbicides, nematocides and plant regulators as defined in the Federal Insecticide, Fungicide and Rodenticide Act.

2. Determining effects of long-term exposure to low levels of pesticides.
3. Regulating and controlling selection, use, transportation and storage of pesticides; and disposal of pesticide wastes to minimize or eliminate direct effects on man or indirect ones through pollution of his environment.
4. Advising consumers at all levels on proper methods for handling, storing, using and disposing of pesticides.

PROBLEMS

Environment Contamination By Pesticides

About 763 million pounds of 900 pesticide chemicals are produced and used annually in the United States for agricultural, industrial, and home purposes. The large scale use of these chemicals poses many problems to Federal, State, and local officials concerned with protection of public health and environment. Significant problem areas include the following:

1. Misuse of approved pesticides by growers, applicators, vector-control programs (i.e., excessive application; selection of wrong formulation, etc.).
2. Accidental contamination of good sources; improperly contained pesticide application, such as wind drift from aerial application; use of contaminated irrigation water, and residues in soil from previous application to other crops.
3. Careless and accidental release of pesticides while in storage or transit. Such incidents lead to contamination of other commodities and are potentially dangerous to man and environment.
4. Improper disposal of waste pesticide chemicals and pesticide containers may contaminate surface, ground and estuarine water and the air or soil.
5. Contamination in formulation and/or packaging of specified pesticides with other pesticides not specified on the label.
6. Pesticide poisoning in the home contributed to 5,739 reported poisoning cases, including 3,965 among children under five years of age. This data is from the Poison Control Centers for 1968, with poisoning defined as ingestion. The number of unreported cases of accidental pesticide poisoning has been estimated at about 15,000 based on 100 poisoning cases for each death reported from all sources. About 12% of the toxic substances most frequently ingested by children under five years of age are pesticides. Pesticides contributed, in large part, to 2,200 deaths from ingestion of hazardous substances. Some 350 of these were children under five. Consumers frequently do not realize or understand the importance of careful handling, use, and storage of these products around the home.
7. Diagnosis and reporting of illnesses and deaths due to exposure to pesticides is far from adequate, thus preventing proper recognition of the problems.

The consequences of acute overwhelming exposure to individual pesticides may be easily recognized. The more subtle effects of long-term, low-level exposure to a variety of pesticides singly and in combination are still to be identified in full and evaluated. Another effect of pesticides to be studied and evaluated is their relationship to the effectiveness of drugs. Unless these effects are properly documented and reported, their true incidence cannot be determined. Community epidemiologic studies may provide leads to the chronic hazard of pesticide exposure from all sources.

8. Overall, there is the problem of contamination of the environment by persistent pesticides which not only affect the ecology but also find their way back into man's food chain. The recent discovery of high levels of DDT in the flesh of Coho salmon taken from the waters of Lake Michigan is illustrative. Low DDT levels in the water were concentrated in the salmon through its food chain and thus presented a potential food product hazard for man. These compounds are also present in potable water and air.

9. Occupational exposure to pesticide chemicals by workers directly involved in manufacture, handling, or application of pesticides is another problem for officials concerned with the protection of the public health. Possible harmful effects to migrant agricultural workers, who commonly work at such jobs as thinning, weeding, or picking, have not been the subject of specific investigation. Residues on crops have, in few instances, caused poisoning in agricultural workers from occupational exposure.

Pesticide Pollution

ARE THE RISKS WELL CALCULATED?

It wasn't until Rachel Carson's "Silent Spring" brought the matter to nationwide attention that the general public realized just how toxic pesticides are and how carelessly they have been used. That book was first published in 1962 by Houghton Mifflin Co. and later made available in a special Consumers Union edition for REPORTS readers. Now, seven years later, the pesticide market continues to boom—despite still-unfolding evidence that the misuse of pesticides may well pose a threat to wildlife, natural systems and man himself. This article, the first of two, reviews some of the reasons why responsible scientists and citizens are concerned about the threat of pesticides. It is a threat that, unfortunately, can only be partially defined. Research on the long-term effects on man is almost completely lacking, and conclusions from research already performed on other animals do not necessarily apply to man. Thus, discussions of possible carcinogenic and mutagenic effects of pesticides on man must, of necessity, be speculative. Still, the number of unexplored risks should be warning enough that continuous monitoring of pesticide dangers demands high national priority. Although the article that follows is not CU's work and we therefore cannot endorse every statement or implication, we feel that it is a valid statement of concern and an effective antidote to apathy. The article itself is an abridged version of a recent CF letter, a periodical published by The Conservation Foundation, an independent, nonprofit group concerned with environmental issues.

Pesticides, complex chemical compounds, pose a complex dilemma. They damage the world's fish and wildlife resources. They are causing serious and subtle changes in the environment. Indeed, they are under suspicion of endangering man himself. Yet man finds them tremendously useful in his struggle for health and survival.

For some 25 years, man has been concocting an astonishing assortment of synthetic chemical poisons and spreading them over the planet. In doing so, he has been taking some not-very-well-calculated risks. He has been rebuked and warned for being careless, for not fully understanding the consequences. Some

Reprinted by permission from *Consumer Reports,* July 1969, pp. 411-413.

restrictions have been imposed; somewhat greater care is being taken. But man continues the liberal use of pesticides to wage war on the endless varieties of insects, bacteria, rodents and other small creatures that continue to plague him so relentlessly—by attacking him directly, or by devouring much of his precious food and fiber supply.

To be sure, the widespread dissemination of pesticides has had extremely tangible benefits which, it is argued, would otherwise have been unattainable. Pesticides are credited with making life comfortable and nuisance-free, indoors and out. They are credited with saving countless lives through the control of malaria, cholera, typhus, Rocky Mountain spotted fever, encephalitis and other diseases. And they are credited with helping man raise and protect an extraordinarily plentiful supply of inexpensive food.

The farm and chemical industries point to the crops and livestock saved from destruction, with values measured in the billions of dollars each year. But the evidence also shows that, in the rush to rely on expedient chemicals, mistakes have been made and safer alternatives have been passed up. There have often been unintended side effects, including losses of fish and wildlife. Finally, the evidence *suggests,* at least, that man may be seriously harming *himself* in the process. Certainly he is taking risks.

How Widely Used?

How extensive is the use of pesticides? U.S. farmers last year spent an estimated $800 million on them. Total domestic sales this year are forecast at $1.7 billion, most for agriculture, but including $255 million for household and garden use, and another $255 million for industrial and institutional use. The $1.7 billion represents a dramatic increase from the 1965 total of $1 billion.

There are some 900 basic chemical compounds used to formulate thousands of synthetic commercial pesticides. Classed according to purpose, these include insecticides, herbicides, miticides, fungicides and rodenticides. Most famous—or infamous—is the ubiquitous DDT. But there are many others endrin, dieldrin, aldrin, chlordane, toxaphene, lindane, methoxychlor, heptachlor, parathion, malathion, 2,4-D, 2,4,5-T, captan, carbaryl, warfarin. There are chlorinated hydrocarbons (DDT), organic phosphates (malathion), and carbamates (carbaryl). Their properties, effects, dosage and use vary widely. The crucial questions raised by the use of a pesticide are: Is it effective on the target insect? What other organisms does it kill? Is it dangerous to fish, wildlife, man?

A pesticide may or may not be highly toxic, or poisonous, on direct contact, to various living things. It may or may not be highly persistent, or resistant to being broken down by nature into harmless components. The insecticide parathion, for example, is extremely toxic. Yet it breaks down quickly in the environment. On the other hand, DDT is considered only slightly toxic to man; but it may persist for years, with consequences unknown.

Some Effects of Pesticide Use

Many ill effects of pesticides on marine life and wildlife are well documented; the literature on the subject is voluminous. A sample of the findings:

Experiments indicate that DDT in very small concentrations can reduce growth and photosynthesis in certain marine plankton. "Such single-celled algae are the indispensable base of marine food chains," says Dr. Charles F. Wurster, Jr., of State University of New York, Stony Brook. Photosynthesis by marine plankton is estimated to account for more than half of the world's oxygen supply. Wurster says that "interference with this process could have profound, worldwide biological implications."

"Marine organisms, especially crustaceans," says William A. Niering, Professor of Botany at Connecticut College, "are extremely sensitive to the persistent pesticides. As little as 0.6 to 6 parts per *billion* (in the water) will kill or immobilize a shrimp population in two days." The Interior Department's Bureau of Commercial Fisheries says tests show that "oysters stopped feeding and exhibited erratic shell movements when exposed to less than one part per million of many chlorinated hydrocarbons. Shell formation in oysters was inhibited by concentrations of a few parts per billion."

Cases in which large numbers of fish have been killed are plentiful. The most celebrated, probably, were the massive kills in the lower Mississippi River from 1960 to 1964. An elaborate investigation traced the cause to endrin, apparently from a chemical plant.

Nearly a million small coho salmon were killed recently because of DDT, say Dr. Howard E. Johnson and Charles Pecor of Michigan State University, who deduced that residues were accumulated in the egg yolk of adults, and their fry were poisoned during final absorption of the yolk sac.

The widespread loss of robins and other birds—where elm trees are treated with DDT for Dutch elm disease—provides a simple example of "biological magnification" or the unique way in which "hard" or persistent pesticides can be concentrated in more and more potent doses as they move up the food chain. When leaves from a sprayed elm fall, they are eaten by earthworms. The DDT doesn't harm the worms; but it accumulates in their tissues. When robins eat the worms, they accumulate it in ever larger and finally lethal doses.

The magnification process also occurs when minute quantities of a pesticide accumulate in tiny marine organisms and are transferred in ever-increasing amounts to plankton-eating fish, carnivorous fish and finally birds of prey. This is possible because pesticides such as DDT are almost totally insoluble in water, but very soluble in fat. So they accumulate and are stored in the fatty tissue of birds. When fat reserves are used up rapidly, such as in migration or reproduction, the poisons enter other parts of the system, apparently attacking the nervous system. Says Dr. Ralph A. MacMullan, director of the Michigan Department of Conservation: There is "strong circumstantial evidence" that this sort of magnification is responsible for the alarming decline of many species of birds such as the bald eagle, osprey, peregrine falcon and sparrow hawk.

Oddly enough, such birds are not normally poisoned directly by the toxic pesticides. It is now widely believed that *reproduction* is severely hampered, because residues of pesticide such as DDT are transferred in lethal amounts to embryo birds via the egg yolk, or because the pesticides upset liver enzyme activity and therefore calcium metabolism, resulting in eggshells so thin embryo chicks cannot survive in them. Studies have also indicated that some birds become strangely nervous and aggressive and destroy their own eggs.

There have been cases in which frogs, snakes and birds, as well as wild and domestic animals, have been killed by pesticides, sometimes in massive numbers. Rachel Carson, in her 1962 best seller *Silent Spring*, cited dozens of instances. Many such kills are due to outright misuse, which of course greatly magnifies the dangers and damage of pesticides. But knowledge, or communication of it to the right people, has not been sufficient to prevent misuse. We do not in fact yet know all the ways in which pesticide applications may be upsetting the balance of nature, though examples from the past are plentiful.

We do know that persistent pesticides are carried throughout the world by wind, water and living organisms. Often cited is the fact that even penguins in the Antarctic—so far from any pesticide use—contain residues of DDT. Dr. George M. Woodwell, an ecologist at Brookhaven National Laboratory, speaks of the "serious and subtle changes caused by continuous exposure to low levels of pesticides in the environment . . . that threatens to degrade the biota of the earth and especially the oceans in a very serious way."

The Dilemma for Man

The weight of expert opinion currently holds that humans are not *directly* harmed by careful use of pesticides. There is apparently no solid evidence of such harm. But practically every human accumulates some pesticides which, as in birds, are stored in body fat. In the U.S. the average is thought to be about 10 to 12 parts per million. Scientists believe that man manages to get rid of pesticide accumulations over a certain level, given a reasonable amount of time. Research on the long-term effects of pesticides on humans is virtually impossible; and it is extremely difficult to extrapolate research on animals to humans. So while there is no convincing evidence that pesticides seriously damage man, neither is there proof that they don't.

A number of scientific studies have linked pesticides and other chemical compounds with cancer. In early March it was reported that preliminary analysis of a large-scale study of 130 such compounds—conducted for the National Cancer Institute—indicates they are carcinogenic to mice (in very large doses). Pesticides are reportedly among the compounds under suspicion.

Other reports suggest that pesticides are a genetic hazard to man, capable of producing mutations, which are usually harmful. Dr. James F. Crow of the University of Wisconsin says, "There is reason to fear that some chemicals [including pesticides] may constitute as important a [mutagenic] risk as radiation, possibly a more serious one." Dr. Osny G. Fahmy of the Chester Beatty Research Institute in London says, "the amount of pesticide chemicals man is now absorbing from his environment is enough to double the normal mutation rate." He says they are capable of disrupting the DNA molecule; the effects are cumulative, and the mutations may not show up for generations. Dr. Marvin Legator of the Food and Drug Administration says the widely used and relatively nontoxic fungicide captan breaks chromosomes in mammalian cell cultures and may be capable of inducing mutations in man. Dr. M. Jacqueline Verrett, also of FDA, says such chemicals can cause birth deformities in chickens. *Medical World News* has reported that a great many genetics experts are concerned about mutagenic chemicals "as either a proved or at least a potential menace to human health . . ."

Dr. Robert W. Risebrough of the University of California's Marine Resources Institute says consideration is not being given to the enzyme-inducing ability of pesticides. "No responsible person could now get up here and say that this constant nibbling away at our steroids (sex hormones) is without any physiological effect. It would be irresponsible."

None of these scientists claims to have *proved* any mass dire effects due to pesticides. But they are warning man that he should not be blind to the possibilities. Man was surprised, after all, when he found that the drug thalidomide could cause children to be deformed; that cigaret smoking could cause cancer; that simple X-rays could cause a skin ailment that didn't show up for decades; or that amounts of radiation presumed to be safe could apparently cause tumors in children more than 10 years later.

Pesticide Poisoning

More obvious are the effects of pesticide poisoning in household, occupational and industrial accidents. "Each year," says a government study, "approximately 150 deaths are attributed to misuse of pesticides in the United States.

About half of these occur in children who were accidentally exposed at home." It would be impossible to guess the number of nonfatal poisonings. But cases of occupational poisoning "have become more frequent," and "the adequacy of safeguards . . . is put in question by reviews of the effects of pesticides on human health."

In California alone in 1964, there were some 1328 reports of occupational disease attributed to pesticides and other agricultural chemicals. This has now become a major new issue in the long, bitter strike and boycott against California's table grape growers. The union argues that many cases of poisoning are not reported, and many others are mistaken for other illnesses because the symptoms are so similar. It has filed suit to halt the use of DDT in the state. In Mexico, 17 were killed and some 600 made violently ill in 1967 when parathion contaminated bread supplies. A week later, a truck loaded with parathion overturned and spilled the deadly pesticide over a California highway.

The Ironies of It All

Aside from misuse and danger, the application of pesticides is likely to be fraught with irony and paradox—in fact, with failure. In the first place, it should be noted that agriculture, particularly in the U.S., has tended to spread single crops over larger and larger areas, sometimes over thousands of acres. Such monoculture is efficient and economical. But it is also an invitation to pests which thrive on a particular crop, especially since their natural enemies may no longer find the area to their liking. Such invitations, of course, have been answered with massive invasions.

Perhaps the greatest irony in pesticide use is the destruction of beneficial insects and rodents in addition to the target species. (There has been some limited success in developing pesticides with narrow, specific effects.) Thus the victims are likely to include the very natural enemies that have been holding the target pest in check. There are many cases in which pest populations have burgeoned anew as a result. Sometimes the destruction of parasites and predators simply clears the field for a surge of *several* new crop pests, compounding the problem of control.

A second is that pests have a perverse tendency to develop resistance to the poisons man lavishes on them. Says a Congressional report: "When a pest population, reproducing rapidly, is exposed to a lethal chemical, the laws of natural selection are dramatically demonstrated. The variety of genetic makeup, even within a single species, means that some insects in the population will have a biochemical mechanism for resistance and a new population will build up, unaffected . . . " Then there is an inclination to increase the dosage, or shift to another perhaps more poisonous chemical, to kill off this tougher breed. But the report cautions that "there appears to be no toxicant powerful enough to kill every member of a large population."

There's another kind of "resistance." For example, Professor Walter Ebeling and Donald A. Reierson of UCLA write of cockroaches that learn to avoid hazardous insecticides even after the first contact, with the result that the most toxic substances may be the least effective.

Metallic Menaces

Gene Bylinsky

Into the already crowded ranks of dangerous pollutants has lately moved a gang of the toughest villains yet—health-impairing metals such as lead, mercury, cadmium, beryllium, nickel, vanadium. Unlike most other pollutants, they are natural substances. Over the years, man has been extracting these metals from stable minerals found in nature and spreading them around in forms that can be harmful. The flow of metallic pollutants into the environment has accelerated in recent decades to such an extent that now the public at large may be threatened with what used to be considered "occupational" health hazards inside mines or factories.

Americans got a disconcerting dose of news about the toxicity and persistence of these contaminants when the mercury scare hit last year. At about the same time, lead additives in gasoline came under an intensifying attack. But many other metallic pollutants are becoming subjects of concern. Beryllium, emitted mainly by processing plants, can damage the respiratory system. So can nickel, which is entering our air from metallurgical plants, from the burning of coal and oil, and as an unburned fuel additive. Cadmium gets into the air through the refining of associated metals such as zinc, lead, and copper. Particles of cadmium are picked up from galvanized water mains and pipes, and so get into our drinking water too. There is evidence that cadmium causes high blood pressure. It can also lead to respiratory ailments and kidney damage. Vanadium, from certain types of fuel oil as well as from refining and alloying, inhibits the synthesis of cholesterol, even in relatively small concentrations. People are now accustomed to think of cholesterol as undesirable, but in small amounts it is essential in metabolism.

This, of course, is far from a complete list. There are twenty or so other metals that bear watching. The special difficulty with all metallic pollutants is their persistence. A man who has done much to call attention to the hazards of metallic pollution, Dr. Henry A. Schroeder of the Dartmouth Medical School, has stated: "Pollution by toxic metals is a much more serious and much more

Reprinted from the January, 1971 issue of *Fortune Magazine* by special permission; © 1971 Time Inc.

insidious problem than is pollution by organic substances such as pesticides, weed killers, sulphur dioxide, oxides of nitrogen, carbon monoxide, and other gross contaminants of air and water. Most organic substances are degradable by natural processes; no metal is degradable."

Little wonder that we are now witnessing the beginnings of restrictions on metallic pollutants. Federal authorities will suggest criteria this year for permissible amounts of lead in the ambient air. Guidelines for beryllium will follow next year. Later on, cadmium, copper, manganese, nickel, vanadium, zinc, chromium, and airborne mercury will come under control. Similar restrictions on disposal of these substances in water are either already in effect or soon will be.

It would be unrealistic, however, to suppose that a complete ban on any of these metals is in the making. They are too essential, too ingrained in our life, too abundant in the natural environment. As one scientist puts it: "We cannot ban metals any more than we can ban the earth." Still, the economic damage from the coming restrictions may prove to be substantial. It may become unprofitable to mine certain ore deposits, for example. And we can expect increasing use of expensive substitute materials where metals might present a health hazard.

IS THERE A "SAFE" LEVEL?

The sudden increase in public awareness of metallic pollution raises a number of serious questions about how society should proceed in weighing potential, and sometimes ill-defined, health hazards against real and immediate economic dislocations. How, for example, can government help smooth over such disruptions? How can it avoid a pseudo-scientific and panicky blacklisting of substances at levels that have always been present around us? How can we determine the "safe" level for a pollutant, or whether there is such a safe level? Says Dr. Harriet Hardy, a respected worker in occupational health: "Great care must be taken not to pass laws that are unenforceable, not only because of economic considerations, but because they are not based on sound data."

The search for sound data about metallic pollutants and their effects encounters a peculiar complication in that metals have been part of the human environment, and the human body, ever since man evolved. No fewer than fifty-one metals, from aluminum to zirconium, are now known to be present in the body in varying amounts. Without some of them, in trace amounts , no plant or animal could live. Iron, magnesium, manganese, molybdenum, calcium, chromium, cobalt, copper, and zinc are known to be essential to life, and vanadium, nickel, and tin are thought to be. Metals, often incorporated into proteins, serve as catalysts that initiate or assist in biological reactions. Each of the four iron atoms in a hemoglobin molecule, for instance, is a "handle" to which oxygen molecules become attached, to be carried throughout the body in the red pigment of the blood. In plants an atom of magnesium serves as the structural hub of every molecule of chlorophyll.

Over the millennia, organisms developed delicate balancing, or homeostatic, mechanisms to regulate the rate at which essential trace metals are incorporated into their tissues. But in general, organisms, including man, failed to develop comparable defenses against the heavier metals that perform no beneficial function. These metals are toxic in their elemental form, especially if they are absorbed as small particles. They become even more hazardous in organic compounds; these are more rapidly absorbed into the body and tend to concentrate in nerve tissue. A notable example is methyl mercury, which is far more dangerous than mercury in its familiar metallic form. Another is tetraethyl lead, which being readily soluble in fats is particularly damaging to nerve centers and to the brain.

THE FALL OF AN EMPIRE

Lead affords a relatively well-documented example of how a metal can be both exceedingly useful and hazardous to health. Like other metals, lead played a vital part in the development of industrial civilization, but absorption of even a small quantity into the human body can cause severe illness. Some scientists have implicated lead in the downfall of the Roman Empire. The Romans, according to some calculations, produced an average of 60,000 tons of lead a year for four hundred years. Some of it went into the making of pots for boiling grape juice to make a syrup used as a preservative and sweetener of wine. This greatly increased the intake of lead, which was also used in cosmetics and medicines. The upshot, the argument runs, was a gradual poisoning of the upper classes (but not of the lower classes, who could not afford as much wine). The poisoning is said to have brought about widespread stillbirths, deformities, and brain damage. One support for this theory is that high lead content has been found in the bones of ancient Romans.

That severe reactions can result from excessive exposure to lead has long been known. Hippocrates described colic in a lead worker. But danger levels weren't determined until the past few decades. Instruments were lacking. Tests on animals can be inconclusive. "Even if we study them to the nth degree," says biochemist Hans Falk, an associate director of the new National Institute of Environmental Health Sciences, "we will never be able to say he's just like Uncle Joe, because he isn't quite." The pioneering research on the danger levels of lead in the blood was done by Dr. Robert A. Kehoe and his associates at the University of Cincinnati's Kettering Laboratory, originally set up with industry funds. In his experiments, Kehoe found no overt poisoning if the initial exposure resulted in lead levels below 80 micrograms (millionths of a gram) per 100 grams of blood.

But there's nothing magic about that 80-microgram line. For one thing, different people respond differently to lead in their blood. Some adults display visible but nonspecific symptoms of poisoning with a blood lead level as low as 60 micrograms, while others remain apparently unaffected with twice as much. In children, symptoms of lead poisoning have been observed at blood lead concentrations of 60 micrograms and suggestions have been made to lower the danger line for children to 40 micrograms. Many experts now consider the 80-microgram standard too high for adults. Some European countries have set the industrial exposure threshold at 70 micrograms.

These yardsticks are only partially useful where exposure of the general public to lead in air, food, and water is concerned. Even in cities, most people encounter much smaller amounts of poisonous contaminants than workers in the metal-producing or using industries. For instance, average lead content of the air of representative U.S. cities, at about 2 micrograms per cubic meter, is only 1/100th of the concentration considered acceptable for industrial plants. But lead concentrations run much higher in dense traffic and in tunnels; concentrations as high as 54 micrograms have been measured in Los Angeles traffic. Most of us, moreover, breathe air with lead in it twenty-four hours a day, instead of the seven or eight hours on which industrial standards are based. Therefore, standards for lead in the ambient air are expected to call for about 2 micrograms per cubic meter. At that rate it would take an average citizen about seventy years to inhale what would amount to approximately a birdshot pellet of lead.

EVIDENCE IN THE ICE

The most tragic examples of non-occupational lead poisoning today occur among children, particularly children who live in slums. The youngsters eat the deceptively sweet flakes of old lead-based paint peeling from walls and windowsills. This problem persists even though paint manufacturers discontinued the use of lead in interior paints about thirty-five years ago. Painting over old paint doesn't help. The walls must be covered by wallboard, and this hasn't been done in many old houses.

Much more widespread, of course, is the threat posed by increasing levels of lead in the air. Surveys of the general population in the U.S. and elsewhere have revealed that concentrations range from about 5 to 40 micrograms of lead per 100 grams of blood, with an average of about 25 micrograms—nearly one-third of the concentration considered dangerous in industrial exposure in the U. S. One scientist has estimated that if it weren't for man's massive use of lead—1,200,000 tons in the U.S. alone each year—blood concentrations would be only 1/100th of the current typical levels. There is no way to know for certain, however, since blood lead levels today are unexpectedly high even among primitive people living far from civilization. There are no "lead-free" people. Even newborn babies have lead in their blood, absorbed from their mothers.

As might be expected, the closer people get to exhaust fumes, the more lead shows up in their blood. In a survey of three cities, published in 1963 by the U.S. Public Health Service, garage mechanics, parking attendants, and traffic policemen showed particularly high concentrations. And people who live near busy highways were shown, in that and subsequent studies, to have more lead in their blood, too. Lead content in the ambient air and in the blood of residents of those three cities—Cincinnati, Philadelphia, and Los Angeles—was recently resurveyed. Analysis of the data will not be completed for some months, but partial results show a 50 percent increase in atmospheric lead in Los Angeles area communities since the first survey.

In the mid-1960's, braving Arctic and Antarctic blizzards, a team led by geochemist Clair C. Patterson of the California Institute of Technology showed how ominously lead concentrations have risen in the air over the Northern Hemishphere. The investigators collected samples of both ancient and more recent ice and snow from near the North and South poles. Many of the samples were obtained from deep tunnels at undisturbed sites.

The lead content of Arctic snow and ice, the scientists found, went up fourfold between 1750 and 1940, and then nearly tripled again since 1940. The first increase reflects the great expansion of lead smelting that followed the industrial revolution, and the second, the use of lead additives in gasoline. In Antarctica, in sharp contrast, the scientists found that the highest levels were one-tenth of those found in the northern snowpack. One reason why not much lead has been deposited in Antarctica yet is that atmospheric circulation is largely confined to the separate hemispheres; also, most of the world's industry is concentrated above the equator.

This rise in the lead content of air in the Northern Hemisphere is reflected in man, too, particularly in bone and soft tissue. These are considered more reliable indicators of accumulated lead than blood because, being a medium of transport, blood mainly reflects the intensity of recent exposure. Comparing lead content in bones of Peruvian Indians who lived six centuries ago with what modern man carries in his bones, scientists found three years ago that Americans had ten times as much lead in their skeletons. The investigators concluded that the increased lead burden is a "striking reflection of modern air pollution." People still take in more lead through their diet (about 300 micrograms a day) than by breathing, but only about one-tenth of the ingested lead is absorbed and retained by the tissues as against at least one-third of the inhaled lead.

Further evidence of a rise in lead deposits in tissue was established a few years ago by physicist Isabel Tipton of Oak Ridge National Laboratory and the University of Tennessee and Dr. Schroeder of Dartmouth. They found that lead accumulates in the tissues of Americans at a far greater rate than in the tissues of Africans living in primitive settings. For example, lung tissue of Americans contained twice as much lead as that of Africans.

LOOKING FOR A DIME UNDER A LAMPPOST

The big unsettled and unsettling question is what the increasing body burden of lead is doing to human health. Early symptoms of lead poisoning are very nonspecific and it can be easily mistaken for any of a number of maladies. The symptoms may include loss of appetite and weight, fatigue, headaches, and anemia. Continued absorption of lead can lead to irritability, lack of coordination, vague pains in the arms, legs, joints, and abdomen. In advanced cases, the victims suffer elevated blood pressure, convulsions, coma, and brain damage.

Given to mice and rats in doses sufficient to reproduce the amount of lead now found in human tissues, the metal has significantly shortened the animals' lifetimes by inducing general weakness and fatigue. Considering the differences in size, this would be a large dose in human terms, of course. But animals respond to smaller amounts of lead, too. Soviet scientists have reported that rats exposed for six hours a day to 11 micrograms of lead per cubic meter of air (or about five times the average concentration in the air of some U.S. cities) showed a slowdown in their conditioned responses—to the sound of a bell, for example—after exposure had continued for three months. After completing the experiments, the scientists found a bit more lead in the rats' bones than people carry in theirs.

No overt symptoms of lead poisoning, such as "wrist drop" caused by neurological damage, have been traced to the levels of exposure that now prevail in the general environment. But looking for such gross symptoms may make as much sense as "looking under a lamppost for a dime you lost a block away," to quote one scientist. If damage is being done to the public at large, it is probably being done very subtly. Dr. Jesse L. Steinfeld, Surgeon General of the U.S., warned recently that a hazard may already exist for people who are particularly sensitive to lead.

TROUBLE IN THE ENZYME SWITCHYARD

Investigation of the effects of low-level lead contamination, therefore, must descend into the deeper, more complex biochemical mechanisms of the body. One of these processes is the synthesis of heme (pronounced heem), the iron-containing component of hemoglobin. This synthesis takes place, in bone marrow and elsewhere, in what might be visualized as a miniature railroad assembly and switchyard. Along a central track, seven switches are operated by seven different enzymes, those busy catalysts of the body's biochemistry. Out of basic building blocks, starting with glycine, the enzymes put together the iron-containing heme train. It is then joined with a protein, globin, to form hemoglobin, the stuff red cells are made of.

A relatively heavy exposure to lead impairs the production of red blood cells. Signs of anemia can be observed in people whose blood lead concentrations hover around that 80-microgram danger line. The evidence for inhibition of heme synthesis by lead goes back as far as 1880, when scientists spotted abnormal amounts of porphyrin—an intermediate of red-cell synthesis—in the urine of people suffering from lead poisoning. It was as if a malfunctioning switch somewhere along that heme assembly line were shunting porphyrin onto a sidetrack.

More recently, another intermediate substance in the making of heme, delta-aminolevulinic acid (ALA), was found in the urine. This discovery suggested interference with the functioning of the enzyme delta-ALA-dehydrase, one of the switchmen in heme synthesis; this enzyme uses ALA to further the production of heme. The ALA starts spilling over from the blood into the urine at lead concentrations of about 50 micrograms, thus providing a "preclinical" sign that excessive exposure to lead has occurred.

The new concern about lead has expanded the search for evidence of damage to the general population. Out of this search came only last year a startling but little noticed report by a group of Finnish researchers. Activity of the enzyme ALA-dehydrase, they discovered, is depressed not only in workers who come in contact with lead, but in everyone. Moreover, the scientists, led by Dr. Sven Hernberg of the University of Helsinki, could find no well-defined level of lead in the blood below which inhibition of ALA-dehydrase did *not* occur.

The Finnish finding, which has been recently confirmed by studies done in the U.S., indicates that at least some degree of biochemical disturbance is taking place in all of us at supposedly normal levels of exposure to lead. But whether depression of ALA-dehydrase activity has any effects on health is not known at present. In most metabolic functions there is usually one "rate-limiting" enzyme that sets the pace for synthesis of a particular substance, and luckily ALA-dehydrase is not rate limiting in heme production. In other words, ALA-dehydrase at what are now considered normal levels of lead in the blood can slow down its work without creating a noticeable effect on red-cell production.

As intake of lead increases, however, it begins to interfere with a number of other enzymes in the synthesis of heme, including the one that *is* rate limiting, ALA-synthetase. Because of this interference with heme synthesis, the 125-day average life span of red cells is reduced in at least some people at the still "normal" level of 60 to 70 micrograms per 100 grams of blood. At 70 micrograms, according to the Finnish study, ALA-dehydrase activity is reduced by about 90 percent. At that point, symptoms of anemia may already be visible.

Heme and its precursors are widely distributed throughout the body, serving in such vital functions as activation of enzymes that control cell respiration. What interests many scientists now is whether formation of heme is being suppressed in some organs of the body beyond these organs' adaptive ability. Last October a group of British scientists reported that activity of ALA-dehydrase is abnormally low in the blood *and* brain of lead-poisoned baby rats. Professor Abraham Goldberg and his colleagues wrote in the *Lancet,* a British medical journal: "It is, therefore, possible that children with blood-lead levels greater than 20 micrograms, in whom there is a significant decrease in blood ALA-dehydrase activity, also have similar decreases in brain enzyme activity."

Such studies, concentrating on young animals and children, on people especially susceptible to anemia, and on thousands of lead workers who may have undetected signs of disease, are expected finally to implicate, or exonerate, prolonged low-level exposure to lead as a cause of ill health. Some scientists think that definite answers should be forthcoming in about five years.

MORE PAINFUL THAN IT SHOULD HAVE BEEN

By then the level of lead in the air should be reduced significantly as a result of the campaign against gasoline additives. Before the recent commotion started, the use of tetraethyl lead to alleviate engine knock had gradually risen to more than 400 million pounds a year to become the No. 1 source of lead in the air. About 80 percent of the lead is emitted from the exhaust as aerosol particles that can penetrate the deep recesses of the lungs.

The rather abrupt and largely unplanned move against lead in gasoline will be economically painful—more so than it should have been. The anti-lead campaign was kicked off in earnest last January not by Ralph Nader but by Edward Cole, president of General Motors, when he said that the auto makers would have a much better chance of coming up with effective exhaust-control devices if lead-free gasoline were available. Researchers had found that a single tankful of leaded gasoline, containing about a teaspoonful of the additive per gallon, can ruin some types of catalytic mufflers, the devices considered most likely to succeed in control of automotive pollution.

The manufacturers of lead additives, for their part, have been arguing that the proposed federal standards for exhaust emissions be met by means of a trap to capture lead and other particles and (instead of a catalytic muffler) a thermal reactor to burn up exhaust pollutants. This line of argument, however, is a last-ditch defense.

Lead is on its way out. Auto makers have now adjusted most of their new cars to run on 91-octane gasoline with reduced lead content, or none at all. To motorists, the change-over to lead-free gasoline will probably mean paying from half a cent to one and a half cents more per gallon, or about $5 to $15 more a year. But, according to a technical panel convened by the Commerce Department, motorists will probably wind up with a saving on maintenance costs because low-lead and lead-free fuels will extend the life of spark plugs and exhaust systems. Complete removal of lead from gasoline could damage valves on some high-compression cars, the panel said, but this problem can be avoided in the future by redesigning the valves.

The adverse economic effect is expected to be felt most acutely by small gasoline refiners, some of which may be forced to shut down, and by lead-additive manufacturers, whose market will gradually disappear. Industry sources estimate that 10,000 workers may lose their jobs. The $400-million-a-year U.S. market for lead additives is dominated by Du Pont and Ethyl, each accounting for an estimated 40 percent. Nalco Chemical Co. and the Houston Chemical division of PPG Industries, Inc., share equally in the remaining 20 percent. Lead additives make up only about 5 percent of Du Pont's nearly $4 billion in annual sales, and the company can be expected to take the ban in stride. "We'll feel this, but we'll survive," an executive says somewhat facetiously.

Since lead additives have accounted in recent years for about 40 percent of Ethyl's total sales and 60 percent of its profits, that company has a much tougher job ahead. President Bruce Gottwald ticks off a number of areas where Ethyl can expand, such as plastics, detergent additives, synthetic alcohols, and chlorinated solvents, but of the struggle over lead he says: "I don't look forward to an outcome with any glee at all."

INTO A TOXICOLOGICAL FIRE

Toxic metals can get into our food, air, or water by devious and unexpected paths. A disturbing case in point has to do with the introduction of nitrilotriacetic acid (NTA) as a substitute for phosphates in detergents. The toxicity of phosphates to people is very low, but they foster the growth of algae in lakes and rivers. NTA alleviates that problem but creates another. Being a chelating, or binding, agent, it can "lock up" metal ions and carry them from metallic surfaces, such as those of water pipes, into the tap water. NTA also may be capable of mobilizing heavy metals such as mercury from lake sediments. The possibility of such dangerous intrusion into environmental processes is leading some scientists to conclude that we may be better off *not* replacing phosphates. Dr. Samuel S. Epstein, a Harvard pathologist, recently summed up the matter before a congressional committee: "Concern for protection of environmental quality is no reason to replace a relatively defined and otherwise controllable ecological problem by potential hazards to human health of undefined dimensions. We may well be jumping from an ecological frying pan into a toxicological fire."

Another unexpected hazard—transformation of a metal into a form much more dangerous than its elemental state—is illustrated by the seemingly sudden emergence of methyl mercury as a potent threat to public health. The "mad hatters" of yesteryear suffered mental instability and tremors as a result of inhaling vapors from metallic mercury, used in processing fur and felt. Today's concern about mercury chiefly has to do with exposure of the public to organic compounds of mercury in fish and other goods. Among these organic compounds, methyl mercury is the worse offender because it can penetrate biological barriers with great ease. Reaching the brain, it can cause insidious damage that may not show up for months or years.

Methyl mercury has been manufactured for some time as a broad-spectrum fungicide for use on seeds. It came as a shock to most scientists, however, when they discovered that nature can make methyl mercury too. Scientists had thought, if they thought about this problem at all, that metallic mercury discharged by industrial plants would sink to the bottom of bodies of water and harmlessly stay there. But anaerobic microorganisms that thrive in sludge on the bottoms of lakes and rivers, where oxygen is limited or completely absent, can transform mercury into methyl mercury. The microorganisms release the soluble compound into the water, and it is then taken up by successively larger organisms. With each upward step in the food chain, methyl mercury becomes more and more concentrated, so that the tissues of some fish high up in the chain show a 3,000-fold concentration compared with the surrounding water.

THE CULPRIT IDENTIFIED

The dangers of methyl mercury first became starkly evident in Japan, where, starting in 1953, more than a hundred people have died or suffered serious neurological damage after eating mercury-contaminated fish. For a number of years the culprit remained unidentified—it was then difficult to detect mercury in minute quantities, particularly in biological specimens. Finally, Japanese scientists pinpointed methyl mercury.

Despite the danger signals from Japan, and later from Sweden, government authorities in the U.S. took no action against methyl mercury for an inordinately long time. Federal researchers found mercury-contaminated shellfish in the badly polluted Houston Ship Channel but failed to follow up. Now that a burst of belated scientific sleuthing is uncovering the dangerous organic compounds of mercury in all kinds of places and organisms, there is danger of exaggerating the hazards. For one thing, the use of better measuring instruments that became available only recently can lead to detection of the metal where it was previously not known to exist. Dr. Schroeder, who observes that "you can always overdo these things," believes that the Food and Drug Administration has been too cautious in setting a limit of 0.5 parts per million on mercury in fish (usually it occurs in the form of methyl mercury). This limit is about 1/100th of the average mercury level in fish in Japanese poisoning incidents, and half the limit set in Sweden—though the Swedes in addition have been cautioned not to eat fresh-water fish more than once a week. Moreover, about 5,000 tons of mercury are estimated to circulate through the global environment each year in the course of natural processes such as erosion from rocks; that is about as much mercury as man introduces into the environment each year. "There has been mercury in fish ever since there were fish," say Dr. Schroeder, "and the same is true of air and water." In some species of ocean fish, natural concentrations are believed to approach the FDA's limit. Last month there was a stir when authorities found concentrations exceeding 0.5 parts per million in some brands of canned tuna. How much, if any, of these levels was a result of man-made contamination? No one could say with any assurance. Still, since it is not clear whether there is a "safe" threshold for organic mercury, it may be better for public-health authorities to err on the conservative side.

THE DIVERSIFICATION RECIPE

Even though exposure to low levels of toxic metals may do no visible damage to healthy adults, there's a possibility of adverse long-range effects on children. Surgeon General Steinfeld said recently that the concern today "is that we do not, by our shortsightedness, condemn future generations to irreversible hazardous health effects." Lead, for instance, is an unerring bone seeker and may be interfering with calcium metabolism in the young. But this possibility has hardly been looked into; it should become an active field of investigation.

A number of other questions should be looked into. We must find out, for example, what is happening to metallic wastes, to see if metals other than mercury can be transformed into highly hazardous chemical states by microorganisms or in some other ways. For highly industrialized countries, such knowledge is vital, particularly for the U.S., which uses about one-third to one-half of the free world's metals. Use of some metals will at least quadruple by the end of this century, multiplying the problems associated with their use. Recycling is obviously the answer, both to avoid pollution and to conserve the metals.

When a ban on a metal's use becomes necessary, we should employ hardheaded planning so as to avoid putting people out of work and companies out of business. Companies can help themselves by avoiding heavy reliance on a single product that is a potential pollutant. That recipe—diversification—also holds for individuals who want to reduce the risks of accumulating metallic and other pollutants. Here, says Hans Falk, the answer is to stick to a well-rounded diet and not rely too much on any single food item such as fish.

There are some hopeful signs, to be sure. Disposal of mercury into U.S. rivers and lakes by industry has now been effectively curtailed. Unfortunately, the mercury already there is not going to go away. It will continue to circulate through food chains, perhaps for centuries, until the organic compounds return to chemically stable forms.

With the merger of some of the splintered pollution control organizations into the newly formed Environmental Protection Agency, there's hope now that much better monitoring of new health hazards will emerge. The President's Council on Environmental Quality will present a plan for such surveillance within the next few weeks. The new monitoring will focus on heavy metals and hazardous organic substances, and will include sampling of our air, water, and food for such contaminants. A worldwild pollution watch under U.N. auspices is being planned, too. It would include utilization of "sentinel" organisms—plants and animals that would be watched for adverse effects of pollutants.

The most hopeful sign is that, out of the current sometimes inept efforts to cope with the new pollutants, there may yet emerge what one scientist calls "a dimension of foresight." That would enable us to meet similar future hazards more effectively, and to spare ourselves and our descendants a great deal of pain, physical and economic.

Cancer Hazards in the Modern Environment

Unlike smoking, which exposes primarily the smoker to cancer risks, contaminants in the atmosphere affect whole populations and are, for the most part, beyond the individual's control. Cancer hazards, of which a few have been identified and many more suspected from epidemiological surveys, tests in animals, or knowledge of chemical structure, are found in air, water, food, and other elements in our living and working conditions. Biological agents, such as viruses, may act alone or in combination with chemicals as cancer-causing factors.

OCCUPATIONAL HAZARDS

The primary objective of studies of occupational cancer-causing agents, of course, is to protect workers whose exposure to high concentrations of carcinogenic chemicals greatly increases their risk over that of the general population. Protective measures include elimination of the agent, and increased use of industrial hygienic practices and techniques for controlling dust and fumes. The intense and long-continued exposure peculiar to a particular occupation provides clues that also assist in pinpointing carcinogenic pollutants present in weak concentrations in the general environment.

Industries concerned with coal tar and its derivatives—pitch, tar oils, and creosote—account for the largest single group of occupational cancers. These materials and other combustion and distillation products of coal, oil shale, lignite, and petroleum caused thousands of cases of skin cancer over the years in many countries. Coal-tar fumes inhaled by workers in coke oven operations, and fogs, mists, and sprays of various oils encountered in oil refineries were implicated in lung cancer. Benzol, a product of the distillation of coal tar as well as a petrochemical, may affect the blood-forming tissues and produce leukemia. Aniline dyes, produced synthetically from substances obtained from coal tar,

Excerpts from *Progress Against Cancer,* A Report by the National Advisory Cancer Council, U.S. Department of Health, Education and Welfare, Public Health Service, National Institute of Health.

were established as a cause of bladder cancer, acting through an intermediate compound, an aromatic amine called 2-naphthylamine.

Various metals and metallic compounds, and minerals, have long been associated with occupational cancer hazards. Nickel compounds were strongly linked with cancer of the nasal sinuses and lung; chromates, iron oxide, radioactive ores, and asbestos, with cancer of the lung; and arsenic with skin cancer. Beryllium has produced a human disease of the lung called berylliosis; several beryllium compounds have produced lung and bone cancers in experimental animals.

In more recent years, arsenic has been implicated in cancer of the lung and several other body sites among copper ore miners, smelters of nickel-cobalt ores, workers in insecticide manufacture, and vineyard workers. Among the latest findings was an observation that smelter workers regularly exposed to arsenic in the atmosphere experienced a rate of lung cancer deaths 3 times higher than did the general population of white men living in the same States. Those with more than 15 years of heavy exposure had an eightfold risk.

Asbestos is a complex and chemically variable fibrous mineral consisting mostly of magnesium-calcium silicate and is widely used in a myriad of industrial products, including asbestos-cement fireproofing, textiles, and insulating materials. It has caused growing concern as a public health hazard. Occupational exposure to asbestos dust has been increasingly associated with a high risk of lung cancer, most frequently in association with a serious lung disease, asbestosis. In one study it was estimated that the average risk of lung cancer among male workers employed for 20 years or more was 10 times that experienced by the general population. Asbestos has been associated occupationally with, and may be a cause of, mesothelioma, a hitherto rare type of malignant tumor of the pleura, the membrane that encases the lungs, or the peritoneum, a similar membrane that lines the abdominal cavity.

Data have been reported showing an increased frequency of lung cancer among asbestos workers who smoked cigarettes. This frequency was greater than that to be expected for a similar population of cigarette smokers who were not asbestos workers.

Results of animal studies have suggested that some types of asbestos may be less hazardous than others and that substitution of these in industrial products may become a practical preventive measure. Such a measure would be important in protecting the whole population, since asbestos is suspected of being also a general environmental hazard because of its use in such varied products as almost all building materials, fireproof theater curtains, brake linings, ironing-board covers, rugs, mail bags, and many others.

Further studies have confirmed an excess risk of lung cancer among uranium miners of the Colorado Plateau; their risk was greater than that of other miners of similar ores without the high radioactivity (randon disintegration products) component. As was the case in asbestos workers, uranium miners appeared to be particularly susceptible to lung cancer if they were smokers of cigarettes.

Another recent example of an occupational hazard was the discovery of an almost fifty-fold increase in lung cancer and other cancers of the respiratory tract among Japanese workers in a mustard-gas factory during World War II. Mustard gas, a poison war gas, is a radiomimetic chemical; it mimics ionizing radiation in its effects on living tissue. The investigation of this correlation followed an unexpected clue that lung cancer discovered in a young man only 30 years old might have been related to his work for 16 months during the War in a mustard-gas factory not far from Hiroshima. During the period 1952 to 1967, investigators located more than 2,500 of the former workers at the factory from 1929 to 1945, or records on them. They identified 33 deaths from cancer of the respiratory tract, compared with an expected number of 0.9. The cancers occurred centrally in the respiratory tract rather than peripherally; they were of the squamous or undifferentiated cell type, and there were no adenocarcinomas.

Dimethylnitrosamine is an industrial chemical that about 10 years ago was linked to cirrhosis of the liver in men occupationally exposed to it. The compound, an effective solvent, is also an intermediate in the production of dimethylhydrazine (the form with an unsymmetrical molecular structure), an important, noncarcinogenic, chemical in the manufacture of drugs and rocket fuels. Studies showed that dimethylnitrosamine was a powerful carcinogen in laboratory animals, capable of inducing malignant tumors of the liver and other visceral organs in rats and other species. Its potency was of such magnitude that minute dosages produced the cancers. Furthermore, about 40 different nitrosamine derivatives subsequently synthesized yielded a variety of tumors in virtually 100 percent of rats given the chemicals either orally or by injection.

Recent findings have suggested that among male chemists in the United States there was an excess of deaths from cancers of the lymph (infection-fighting) organs and the pancreas. These results came to light in a study of the causes of death among members of the American Chemical Society over a 20-year period and suggest that chemical carcinogens may have a role in the origin of cancers of these sites.

Among the occupationally related cancers unknown in the United States is bladder cancer in Egypt among peasants who work in the waters of the Nile infested with a fluke, *Schistosoma haemotobium*. The parasite enters the body through the skin, and eventually encysts itself in the bladder wall, producing chronic changes that may terminate in cancer. It is not known whether this parasite secretes a chemical substance, or carries a virus, or acts as a cocarcinogen permitting localization in the bladder of unidentified carcinogens contained in the diet of the people.

GENERAL BACKGROUND POLLUTION

Pollution of air and water is one of the great national problems of today. Air pollution obliterates the skyline in cities and destroys natural and man-made beauty. It damages fabrics, metals, and building materials; it kills plants and causes disease in animals. Air pollution is linked with asthma, bronchitis, emphysema, heart disease, the common cold, and cancer—particularly lung cancer. It caused widespread illness and an increased number of deaths among inhabitants of the Meuse Valley, Belgium, in 1930; Donora, Pennsylvania, in 1948; and London, England, in 1952. These resulted from severe local conditions that prevented normal movement and dissipation of pollutants in the air.

Composite data from New York State, Connecticut, and Iowa showed that, generally, cancer occurred more frequently in urban than in rural populations. Among men, the rates for city dwellers were higher especially for cancer of the lung and other parts of the respiratory system, and esophagus. A slightly smaller urban-rural difference was observed for women than for men, especially in the digestive and respiratory systems.

The incomplete combustion of organic matter and fuels from industrial sources, automobile exhausts, incinerators, and other inventions of modern living has introduced into the atmosphere high concentrations of polycyclic aromatic hydrocarbons, such as benzo (a) pyrene. Studies showed that some of this group of compounds are carcinogenic (in animals) and some noncarcinogenic, and that individual hydrocarbons exert inhibitory as well as enhancing effects on one another when present in different amounts. Agents of a different chemical nature occur in the atmosphere also. These may act as cocarcinogens or may otherwise affect the action of polycyclic aromatic hydrocarbons. Noncarcinogenic chemicals (such as phenols) and biological agents in polluted air also may affect the biological action of carcinogens.

Contamination of water supplies with all kinds of products of industrial and individual use is increasing. Recently detergents and insecticides have received particular attention. In southern United States, around the delta of the Mississippi, the inhabitants are susceptible to a high frequency of bladder and lung cancers not entirely attributable to industrial exposure or tobacco smoking. One study about 10 years ago reported an occurrence rate for bladder cancer that was three times higher in New Orleans than in each of two other southern cities, Birmingham, Alabama, and Atlanta, Georgia. Contaminated drinking water was suspected as a potential source of the trouble; laboratory studies to date have not yielded supportive evidence. Purification of water systems, chemically as well as bacteriologically, is one of the great challenges facing the United States.

Another important background environmental carcinogen is physical energy from ionizing radiation and ultraviolet rays. Fair-skinned people exposed to intense ultraviolet radiation from the sun are clearly at higher risk of skin cancer than are others. Skin cancer occurs most frequently in the southern belt of the United States from New Mexico to the Atlantic coast. The relationship is even more striking in Australia, where solar radiation is more intense than in most areas in the United States. Increased skin pigment protects against this type of cancer.

The most convincing evidence that ionizing radiation can induce human leukemia was obtained in studies of the survivors of the atomic bombs in Hiroshima and Nagasaki, and of other groups exposed to relatively large amounts of whole-body irradiation in nuclear accidents. Between 1947 and 1958 the incidence of leukemia in the atomic bomb survivors was 10 times higher than that expected in the population under ordinary circumstances. Other studies have shown that exposure of children to ionizing radiation directed to the nose and throat or to the chest has increased the occurrence of cancer of the thyroid and other sites.

On the other hand, not as much is known about the effects of small doses of irradiation, such as those from natural "background radiation" from rocks and soils, and fallout from nuclear tests. Radioactive fallout begins within hours after an explosion in the atmosphere and may continue for years, although the largest fraction comes to earth within the first year. Strontium-90 and cesium-137 are the fallout products of major importance; both are elements with long half-life and are readily absorbed into the body. In recent years, other test techniques have been introduced, such as underground explosion of atomic weapons.

POLLUTANTS IN EDIBLE MATERIALS

One of the most important and difficult public health problems is that of possible risks due to food additives and contaminants, such as pesticides; and drugs, such as oral contraceptives. The Food and Drug Administration, in the Department of Health, Education and Welfare, has some jurisdiction over these, and the Department of Agriculture also has some responsibility.

With respect to possible cancer risk, addition is prohibited by law of any amount of any chemical that produces cancer when ingested by man or animals. However, the decision of what is or is not cancer producing is based on interpretation by a technically qualified commitee of the results of complex tests in large numbers of animals, usually mice and other species, at several dose levels, and by varying routes of administration. The Department of Health, Education, and Welfare has responsibility for ruling on the carcinogenicity of an additive, such as a food coloring substance, and for enforcing such a ruling.

Pesticides may be hazardous to man either because they persist in trace amounts on the surface of plants or are incorporated into the tissues of plants or animals used by man as a source of food. Under the provisions of the Federal Food, Drug, and Cosmetic Act, such substances must be proved safe by the manufacturer before they may be used. Limits are set by the Food and Drug Administration for the amount of pesticide chemicals that may remain on or in raw agricultural products without harm to the consumer; the Department of Agriculture approves the usefulness of such chemicals and registers them. The tolerances are established on the basis of chemicals present in or on raw foods as shipped in interstate commerce. With respect to a cancer risk, it has been determined that the legislation mentioned above may also be applied to such residues of agricultural chemicals that remain on raw agricultural products.

An example of a compound that did not get into commercial use was N-2-fluorenylacetamide (also known as 2-acetylaminofluorene), which is an effective insecticide. Acute toxicity determinations showed that it was harmless to rats, mice, and rabbits; but the chronic toxicity tests showed the compound to be a potent carcinogenic agent. It evoked a wide spectrum of cancers—of the liver, breast, bladder, and several other sites. This compound today is one of the most widely studied in the laboratory for information on the mode of action of carcinogens in the body.

In May 1963 the President's Science Advisory Committee issued a report on the "Use of Pesticides," recommending additional studies on "Chronic effects on organs of both immature and adult animals, with particular emphasis on tumorigenicity." In response to this need, the National Cancer Institute undertook long-term studies of the toxic effects of a number of pesticides and other agricultural and industrial chemicals, some of which are in wide use. These complex investigations, begun in 1964, constituted the largest group of such experiments performed in a single effort and involved approximately 20,000 mice and 130 chemical compounds. The substances were tested at their maximum tolerated doses, enormously higher than any to which human beings would ever be exposed. The results of the study are being carefully analyzed and evaluated.

A preliminary report in early 1969 on 120 of the compounds showed that under the conditions of high doses administered orally, 11 compounds were tumorigenic for the two strains of mice under study; 89 compounds showed no tumorigenicity; and 20 gave inconclusive results and required further evaluation. The active compounds included five insecticides, such as DDT (a chlorinated hydrocarbon), five fungicides, and a herbicide. The tumors obtained were principally those of the liver, and also tumors of the lung and lymphoid organs.

Interpretation of the results for the purpose of extrapolating them with reference to man is hindered by a lack of important information, including the effect of the chemicals in other species of animals, improved criteria for determining whether the tumors were malignant or benign, and determination of the tumor-inducing role of individual compounds as compared with that of complex chemical mixtures, which might simulate the environmental exposure of man. The National Cancer Institute is continuing its close collaboration with both Federal and other scientists, and others concerned, to obtain the answers to these questions as rapidly as possible.

Another action taken on April 21, 1969 to protect the public from the hazards of pesticides was the appointment by the Secretary of Health, Education, and Welfare of a Commission on Pesticides and their Relationship to Environmental Health. Its charge was to focus on the pesticide DDT and others which, once introduced, become a permanent feature of the environment, and to report back with specific suggestions for action in 6 months.

On November 11, 1969, the Commission submitted preliminary recommendations in support of several basic principles. These suggest that chemicals, including pesticides used to increase food production, are so important in modern life that we must learn to live with them; that the value of chemicals must be individually judged; and that scientific data about their effects on total environment must be accumulated. It was also recommended that final judgments regarding use of such chemicals must be made by the government agencies responsible, by law, for pesticide registration and protection of public health.

Studies have shown that the average person in the United States has 12 parts per million of DDT in his fatty tissue. Concern has centered on the finding that fish in many parts of the country also have significant levels of the pesticide in their tissues, as do red meat supplies and milk.

There is no definite evidence at this time of an adverse effect on man at the concentrations of DDT observed. However, the Food and Drug Administration early in the year established an "interim" tolerance of five parts per million of DDT in the edible parts of fish shipped in interstate commerce. About 90 percent of the fish marketed in this country does not contain residues exceeding one part per million. Late in November the Secretary of Agriculture took stops to ban most uses of DDT by the end of 1970. A number of States had already banned or were considering banning the use of this pesticide.

The ubiquitous polycyclic aromatic hydrocarbons, produced in the incomplete combustion of organic materials and identified as occupational hazards, carcinogens in cigarette "tar," and atmospheric pollutants, are suspected also as contaminants of a wide variety of foods. It is suspected that other carcinogenic organic products may be produced under certain circumstances during the cooking or processing of certain foods.

The well known potent hydrocarbon carcinogen, benzo (a) pyrene, has been found in smoked foods, charcoal-broiled steaks, bread, and roasted coffee beans. Its presence in home-smoked foods was as much as 20 times higher than in factory-smoked products, in a study of the high death rate from stomach cancer in Iceland. The results supported evidence of a relationship between stomach cancer and consumption of home-smoked and singed foods, which contained more polycyclic aromatic hydrocarbons than the commercial products.

Another class of suspected carcinogens consists of the so-called "natural" products or metabolites of various forms of life, such as molds and fungi. Mycotoxins, poisons elaborated by molds and fungi, are represented particularly by the aflatoxins, metabolic products of *Aspergillus flavus.* The aflatoxins are toxic and carcinogenic to the liver when included in the diet of test animals, such as rats. But when injected subcutaneously, these substances cause local sarcomas (solid connective tissue tumors).

A toxic strain of *Penicillium rubrum,* another source of mycotoxins, has been isolated, and it, too, is poisonous to the liver. In Japan, yellow rice was found to be contaminated by a mycotoxin produced by a strain of the *Penicillium islandicum.* It was toxic to the liver of rats and mice, and carcinogenic to rats fed large amounts of rice extract. Two liver-toxic substances were isolated from contaminated rice, but their cancer-inducing activity has not yet been established.

In another study recently reported in Japan, certain popular fermented foodstuffs consumed daily and in quantity by almost everyone were investigated to find possible toxic agents that might be related to the high frequency of stomach cancer among these people. The foodstuffs included "miso," or fermented soy bean paste, and "katsuobushi," or fermented dry bonitos (a type of fish). Numerous strains of fungi were isolated, many of which were found to produce toxic culture filtrates and extracts. None produced aflatoxin. Biologic tests carried out with the culture preparations revealed the development of miscellaneous pathologic changes. The changes in the stomach and liver of animals were of particular interest because of the high incidence of human gastric and liver diseases observed in epidemiological surveys.

An example of a cancer-inducing plant component is cycasin, present in the cycad nut. Extracts of plants containing toxic chemicals called pyrrolizidine alkaloids, have been used in many parts of the world as folk medicines and in rituals. Many livestock losses have been attributed to these substances. It is suspected that "bush teas" containing these alkaloids may have contributed to a high incidence of diseases of the liver, including tumors, observed in natives in certain areas such as the part of Africa south of the Sahara.

It has been suggested that a carcinogen is present in food or beverages, such as herb teas, used in Transkei in South Africa, and the Island of Curacao in the Caribbean, where esophageal carcinoma occurs frequently among the natives. Some of the most frequently used herb teas are being tested in laboratory animals—aqueous extracts of Curacao plants such as mampuritu, kalbas, mango, and passiflora added to the drinking water of mice proved weakly carcinogenic, and are being tested further in more concentrated form.

Safrole, a flavoring agent that is the chief constituent of oil of sassafras, is another type of carcinogen found in plants. Until evidence was obtained that it produced liver tumors in rats when given in the diet in high doses, safrole was used in small amounts to flavor root beer and sarsaparilla. A derivative, dihydrosafrole, proved carcinogenic for the esophagus but not for the liver of the rat.

Sodium cyclamate, an artificial sweetener, came under suspicion as a possible danger to human beings when large doses given to animals were found to yield a breakdown product, cyclohexylamine, which damages chromosomes. Other studies have recently shown that sodium cyclamate causes bladder cancer in rats. These findings led the Secretary of Health, Education, and Welfare to announce a restriction of cyclamates to use in foods and as a sugar substitute, a ban on use of the sweetener in diet beverages by January 1970, and approval of the labeling of food products to show the amount of cyclamates in an average serving; he also emphasized that cyclamates should not be consumed indiscriminately.

Among drugs, those that have received the most attention with respect to possible cancer-inducing activity have been certain hormonal agents used as oral contraceptives. The relationship of hormones to cancer was one of the earliest areas of interest in cancer research. In laboratory animals, the origin of tumors of several organs—breast, ovary, testicle, and pituitary—has been associated with hormonal factors. But no unequivocal evidence is available to support the concept that human cancer may arise as a prime consequence of the normal production of any hormone.

Recent animal studies have suggested that cancer of the uterine cervix was induced in mice by long-term administration of an anti-fertility drug used for human birth control. The drug contained a type of female sex hormonal compound known as a progestational agent. Long-term studies are in progress to determine whether there is a link between the use of oral contraceptives and human cervical carcinoma. In the meantime, the Advisory Committee on Obstetrics and Gynecology of the Food and Drug Administration has recommended regular examination at 6- or 12-month intervals of women using these compounds, and repeated examination of the breasts and cytological study of cervical specimens ("Pap" test).

Evidence is accumulating that use of oral contraceptives increases the risk of some types of thromboembolic disorder (blocking of blood vessel by a clot). Several epidemiologic studies have revealed a risk three to seven times higher among women taking oral contraceptives than among others matched by age, marital status, and other factors.

There is no firm evidence that female sex hormones of the estrogenic type have induced cancer in doses normally given in the clinic. It has been recommended that when estrogens are given at the time of menopause, the dose should be kept small enough for the liver to be able to inactivate it and that administration should be intermittent rather than continuous.

In general, in making decisions as to whether to prescribe a drug, the physician weighs the risk against the beneficial effects. Not only is the cancer hazard a consideration, but also the acute and chronic toxic effects. Large-scale epidemiologic studies, some already under way, should point up the hazards that may attend administration of drugs such as hormones for contraceptive and other purposes. Results of such studies will assist the physician in making decisions for treatment of specific patients.

VI. UNDERSTANDING PEOPLE

POLLUTION

Population, Growth, and Resources

As population grows, it creates more environmental problems and intensifies those that are already there—just by dint of its growth. For all the decades of the country's national existence, population growth has been in a steady spiral. As it grew, there were more people to want more services, which can only come from natural resources. In those nearly two centuries of growth, Americans took what they wanted with little counting of the cost in natural resources and the toll this took on the environment.

We have wanted automobiles, TV sets, and household appliances and a variety of clothing, food, and housing. We have wanted to flip on a switch and immediately have electricity or to turn on a faucet and have an unlimited flow of water at low cost. And we have wanted to dispose easily and rapidly of personal, household, and industrial wastes produced by our style of living.

POPULATION AND GROWTH

Between 1830 and 1930 the world's population doubled from 1 to 2 billion. By 1970, it had almost doubled again, reaching 3.6 billion. Between now and the end of the century, a mere 30 years, it probably will more than double again—barring catastrophe or a marked change in values—to an estimated 7.5 billion. The U.S. population is growing less rapidly than that of most of the rest of the world, but the increase is still significant. One hundred million people lived in the United States in 1915. The population has passed 205 million today and may reach between 265 and 322 million by the end of the century.

Population growth was of little relevance and of no concern to man during the first several hundred thousand years of his existence. Less than 200 years ago, some of the negative implications of population increase first began to be realized.

Although the rate of population growth in the United States and other industrial nations has declined, its absolute growth hasn't. And that contributes

Reprinted from *Environmental Quality,* The First Annual Report of the Council on Environmental Quality, Transmitted to the Congress, August 1970.

to environmental decay. More people mean more congestion, more urban sprawl, and vast networks of highways to transport them. They require more goods and services—more steel, more paper, more cars, and more beer cans. And they put more severe demands on urban land. Moreover, people themselves produce waste that must be handled by treatment plants.

Mushrooming population growth doesn't necessarily mean more polluted air and water. But it is more difficult to have environmental quality with the pressure of population. It is more difficult to avoid congestion, preserve green space and keep a pleasant environment. Whatever the environmental problem, rising population requires effort just to stand still and great effort to make progress—requiring institutions not now available and management tools not yet perfected . . .

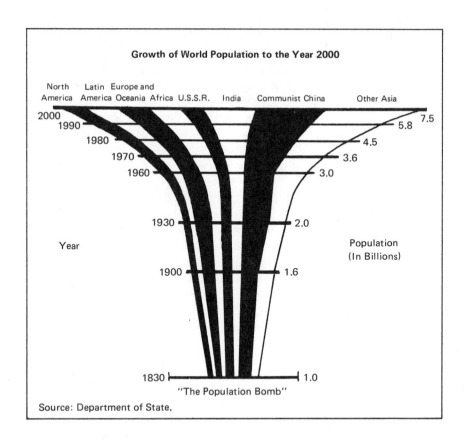

Growth of World Population to the Year 2000

Source: Department of State.

Realities of the Population Explosion

Phillip F. Low

In 1798 Thomas R. Malthus, an English economist and clergyman, published a book entitled *Essay on the Principle of Population.* The main idea of the book was that population tends to increase more rapidly than food supplies, and that, unless war and pestilence killed people off, there would be starvation.

Malthus's dire prediction has been rejected and revived many times. Today it is being revived again. The neo-Malthusians are currently claiming that the population of the world is increasing so rapidly that extreme measures should be taken by governments to curtail population growth. Not only will we run out of food, they say, but we will also exhaust other natural resources, suffer unbearable pollution, experience more war and crime, have so much congestion in our cities that life cannot be enjoyed in them, have inferior social services, and experience a general deterioration in the quality of life. They strongly advocate birth control by contraception, sterilization, abortion, and the imposition of a special tax upon those who have more than a specified number of children, usually two.

A sample of this idea is taken from a letter to the scientific journal *Science.* In the March 13, 1970, issue, Gerald Gelber writes, after referring to two methods of birth control, "Some might say that both alternatives smack of thought control, deprivation of personal liberties, and moral evil. Of course, they are correct. Consider the final alternative: total economic collapse and demoralization of earth's population within two or three generations!"

And in an editorial in the July 31, 1970, issue, Garett Hardin concludes: "If parenthood is a right, population control is impossible. If parenthood is only a privilege, and if parents see themselves as trustees of the germ plasm and guardians of the rights of future generations, then there is hope for mankind."

Yet there are other voices that are less anxious. Ansley J. Coale, after presenting a very logical discussion on population growth in relation to the environment, writes, "To design policies consistent with our most cherished social and political values will not be easy, and it is fortunate that there is no

Reprinted by permission from *The Ensign,* 1, No. 5: May 1971.

valid reason for hasty action."[1] Dr. Coale is director of the Office of Population Research at Princeton University. . . .

As an introduction, it is important to know that it is difficult, if not impossible, to make accurate predictions about the population levels of the future. This is because the factors that control population do not remain constant. Thus, if one extrapolates the trend in the United States birthrate between 1957 and 1968 (see Table 1) into the future, the birthrate will be zero in only about twenty-two years. Obviously, this is ridiculous. If the trend in birthrate between 1919 and 1936 had been extrapolated into the future, the prediction would have been that birth in the United States would cease altogether by 1975.[2] Again, this is ridiculous. Therefore, caution should be exercised in forecasting future populations.

Table 1. Birthrate in the United States by Year				
Year	Birthrate (No. per 1000 persons)	Year	Birthrate (No. per 1000 persons)	
1910	30.1	1960	23.7	
1915	29.5	1961	23.3	
1920	27.7	1962	22.4	
1925	25.1	1963	21.7	
1930	21.3	1964	21.0	
1935	18.7	1965	19.4	
1940	19.4	1966	18.4	
1945	20.4	1967	17.8	
1950	24.1	1968	17.5	
1955	25.0	1969	17.7	

Source: Statistical Abstract of the United States, 1970.

Bar chart values: 30.1, 27.7, 21.3, 19.4, 24.1, 23.7, 19.4, 17.7 for years 1910, 1920, 1930, 1940, 1950, 1960, 1965, 1969.

The Problem in the United States

Let us consider first the population problem in the United States. Here is where the greatest excitement is. Note that Tables 1 and 2 show the birthrate is declining rapidly; yet population is increasing with phenomenal rapidity. Not

Table 2. Population of the United States for the Years 1790 to 1970

Year	Population (millions)	Year	Population (millions)
1790	3.93	1890	62.95
1800	5.31	1900	75.99
1810	7.24	1910	91.97
1820	9.64	1920	105.71
1830	12.87	1930	122.77
1840	17.07	1940	131.67
1850	23.19	1950	150.70
1860	31.44	1960	178.46
1870	39.82	1950	151.33[1]
1880	50.16	1960	179.32
		1970	210.30[2]

Source: Statistical Abstract of the United States, 1967.
[1]Figures above here exclude Alaska and Hawaii.
[2]Obtained from August 31, 1970, issue of *U.S. News and World Report.*

long ago the U.S. Census Bureau projected four different birthrates.[3] The one that was next to the lowest predicted a population of around 308 million by the year 2000, compared to around 200 million today. However, an analysis of the 1970 census in *U.S. News and World Report* for August 31, 1970, indicated that this figure must be revised downward. The same conclusion was reached by the National Goals Research Staff established in 1969 by President Richard M. Nixon.[4] This advisory group suggests that the population might well be stabilized (that is, have zero growth rate) by the year 2000. (Other demographers seem to think likewise.) If the death rate stays at about 9.5 per thousand (Table 3) and the trend in birthrate (Table 1) continues, such a possibility is not hard to visualize.

Reasons for Population Control

1. *Food.* Let us consider some of the factors that are supposed to warrant population control in the United States. One is the potential lack of food. About 1935, a yield takeoff (or sudden increase) occurred in the United States for all grains. Since that time the yield per acre has climbed steadily upward. Speaking of this phenomenon, one expert has said, "Once

Table 3. Birth and Death Rates by Country

Country	Year	Birthrate[1]					Death Rate[2]
USA	1969	17.7					9.5
Argentina	1967	22.3					8.7
Australia	1968	20.0					9.1
Belgium	1969	14.6					12.4
Canada	1969	17.6					7.3
China (Taiwan)	1969	25.6					5.3
France	1969	16.7					11.3
India	1951-61	41.7					22.8
Israel	1969	26.1					6.8
Italy	1969	17.6					10.1
Japan	1969	18.3					6.7
Mexico	1969	42.2					9.1
Netherlands	1969	19.2					8.3
Pakistan	1965	49.0					18.0
Peru	1967	31.9					7.6
Sweden	1969	13.5					10.4
USSR	1968	17.2					7.7
United Kingdom	1969	16.6					11.9

Source: Statistical Abstract of the United States, 1970.
[1]Number of births per 1000 persons.
[2]Number of deaths per 1000 persons.

underway, yield takeoffs appear to be irreversible except in time of war or some similar disaster. Thus far, all have continued indefinitely—the rising yield trends have not leveled off or shown any tendency to level off. If anything, the rate of yield incease tends to accelerate as a country becomes more advanced."[5] The cause is scientific research in agriculture. And there is no reason to believe that research will not continue to produce new technological advances. Also, millions of acres of our arable land are being held in reserve and could be used, along with millions more of marginal land, for food production. Few agronomists that I know would contend that the United States is in danger of a shortage of quality food in the foreseeable future.

2. *Pollution.* Another factor that is supposed to dictate against further population growth is pollution. But, as noted by Henry Wallich, "Per square mile, our [U.S.]population is minimal compared with that of European countries which seem to be able to maintain reasonable standards of public cleanliness, decorum, and social efficiency.

   "If large parts of our country are polluted, it is not because we are too numerous, but because we pollute. The way to stop that disgrace is not to stop having children, but to start cleaning up. The growth of the GNP, sometimes now referred to as gross national pollution, gives us the resources for the job."[6]

3. *War and Crime.* As regards war and crime, it is likely that overcrowded conditions are conducive to aggressive and criminal behavior. Hitler claimed that he moved eastward into Poland for *lebens-raum* (living space). However, these conditions are not the basic cause of crime. If they were, the most crowded areas of the world would be expected to have the highest crime rates. As noted by T. C. Jermann, this is not so.[7] The Netherlands, for example, with the highest overall population density in the world (Table 4), has one of the lowest crime rates in the Western world. And while England has fifty million people crowded into an area smaller than California, there are fewer murders in the entire British Islands every year than in Chicago or Cleveland. Population density, in itself, does not produce crime.

4. *Natural Resources.* Insofar as the exhaustion of natural resources is concerned, the recycling of some of these, such as our mineral resources, is plausible and would certainly minimize the rate of their depletion. Some of the minerals in obsolete airplanes, automobiles, refrigerators, and other equipment and machinery could be reclaimed and used again. On the other hand, it is impossible to recycle fossil fuels such as coal and oil. Ultimately they will be exhausted. But nuclear energy, as a source of power, is being developed rapidly. There is a limitless supply of nuclear energy, and it will likely be possible to operate nuclear power plants with no air pollution, few radiological hazards, and even little thermal pollution. An optimistic article in this regard was recently written by Alvin N. Weinberg, director of the Oak Ridge National Laboratory, U.S. Atomic Energy Commision.[8] He visualizes that nuclear energy can supply the energy needs of the world without creating insoluble problems of pollution, even if its population reaches twenty billion. He also visualizes the use of nuclear energy to desalinize seawater and to extract minerals from low-grade ores that are currently unusable. Consequently, the supply of natural resources need not be a critical factor in limiting population growth.

5. *Congestion.* We do have congested cities. Here, the basic problem is one of

Table 4. Annual Rate of Change and Density of Population for Selected Countries

Country	Annual Rate of Change (1963-68) (%)	Population Density[1] (No. per sq. mi.)
United States	1.2	55
Argentina	1.5	23
Australia	1.9	5
Belgium	0.7	819
China (mainland)	1.4	198
China (Taiwan)	2.9	972
France	0.9	237
East Germany	-0.1	409
Germany, F. R. of	0.9	627
India	2.5	416
Israel	2.9	346
Japan	1.1	710
Netherlands	1.3	985
USSR	1.1	29
United Kingdom	0.6	590
World	1.9	68

Source: Statistical Abstract of the United States, 1970.

[1]Figures for 1968.

The Large squares represent one square mile. Each small square represents a population density of 10 persons per square mile.

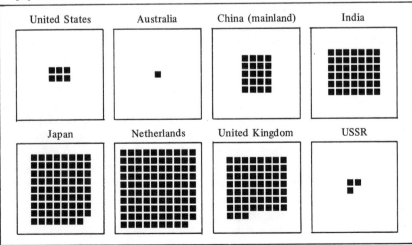

United States   Australia   China (mainland)   India

Japan   Netherlands   United Kingdom   USSR

population distribution. According to *U.S. News and World Report* for August 31, 1970, more than half the nation's 3,042 counties lost population in the 1960s. There are some villages in New England with smaller populations now than at the time of the Civil War. The trend toward the cities has been going on for a long time. It is estimated that by the year 2000 twelve metropolitan areas will occupy one-tenth of the land area in the United States but will contain over seventy percent of the population.

What is needed is a redistribution of the population. This fact is admitted by President Nixon's National Goals Research Staff. They call attention to three ways of achieving it: Spread population by generating growth in sparsely populated rural areas, foster the growth of existing small cities and towns in nonmetropolitan areas, and build new cities outside the large metropolitan regions. In an article in the *Improvement Era* (December 1969, pp. 11-14), Dr. Athelstan Spilhaus, president of Philadelphia's Franklin Institute, is quoted as saying, "If cities with a population of some 250,000 each were scattered evenly across the U.S., we would not have the population problems, traffic problems, riots, and many other ills that develop when cities become too large." It is also noted that he believes pollution comes from concentration, and that if the population were dispersed across the land in small cities, there would probably be no pollution problems. Then it is pointed out that his ideas are similar to those of Joseph Smith, who envisioned small cities of 15,000 to 20,000 surrounded by a green belt and with many other attractive features. His ideas, as described in the article, could be commended to modern city planners.

Those who believe that population control is the universal panacea for all of our problems seem to be unaware of the alternative solutions that have been proposed. They also seem to be unaware that population control has its negative aspects. Let's consider some of these.

For zero population growth to occur immediately in the United States, as some want, it would be necessary to cut the birthrate about in half. We have a young population because of our past history of high birthrates. Thus, a large proportion of the population is concentrated in ages in which the mortality is small. To bring the birthrate down to equal the death rate, women would, for the next fifteen to twenty years, have to bear children at a rate that would produce only a little over one child per completed family. At the end of that time, there would be a very peculiar age distribution with a great shortage of young people. This would bring economic and social disruption.

In a growing population, there is a correspondence between the diminishing numbers of people at higher ages and the diminishing number of leadership positions. In a stationary population, with its uniform distribution of ages, there would no longer be a reasonable expectation for advancement as one grows older. This would kill incentive.

Another argument against zero population growth is that, as noted earlier, the proportion of older people is increased. Consequently, the burden of pensions increases; there is more sickness, and hence, more need for nursing homes, hospitals, and medical care; there is decreased adaptability to changing technology; and there is less innovation and greater conservatism. Further, the economy tends to stagnate. It is fear of economic stagnation, or at least of economic slowdown, that has motivated Japan, the most densely populated country on earth, to adopt a policy to increase its birthrate. As of 1968, Japan had 3,508 people per square mile of *cultivated* land, compared with 1,487 per square mile in runner-up Holland. Some Japanese economists maintain that a decline in West Germany's economic growth rate in the late 1950's was caused primarily by a drop in the growth rate of Germany's work population, and they suggest that Japan's economic miracle may be stalled by the same problem.

Regardless of the ethics of certain groups within the United States, family planning will probably become increasingly popular. And as research in contraceptive methods continues, more effective and convenient means will be discovered. Also, it is not improbable that abortion will be legalized in many states. Already twelve states have reformed their abortion laws, four have declared their abortion laws unconstitutional, test cases are pending in others, and in New York State, abortion is a private matter between the doctor and his patient. All of this will have an impact on population growth, especially since statistics reported in *Science* show that, on the average, 20 percent of all births are unwanted.[9]

It is to be genuinely hoped, and we should exert our influence to see that this hope is realized, that we are permitted to enjoy freedom of choice as enunciated in the 1966 United Nations Declaration of Population: "The opportunity to decide the number and spacing of children is a basic human right."

But some would have it otherwise. In the *Congressional Record* of August 11, 1970 (vol. 116, no. 138), the Honorable John G. Schmitz reports that in the state of California a bill to remove all state income tax deductions for more than two children has been approved by the Revenue and Taxation Committee of the state senate. In the United States Congress, legislation has been introduced in both the House and the Senate to remove the federal personal income tax deductions for all children after the second. And in Hawaii a bill before the state legislature would compel the sterilization of all women after they have their second child. Then he states, "Such legislation heralds the coming of a new Nazism to our land."

It was hopeful to read in *Newsweek*, January 25, 1971, an opposing viewpoint: "Last week no less an authority than the government's chief demographic expert attacked the conventional wisdom head-on and offered an entirely different view of the effects of overpopulation. 'Economic and social factors are more important than population growth in threatening the quality of

American life,' declared Conrad F. Taeuber, supervisor of the 1970 census, in a speech delivered at Mount Holyoke College. 'The population problems of the United States are and will be much more a matter of geographic distribution and the way we use our resources than of the rate of increase in our total numbers.

" 'Changing standards and habits, in activities, technology and the style of life have much more to do with the accumulation and disposition of waste materials and pollutants than does the number of persons involved.' While the U.S. population increased 13 per cent in the last decade, the total volume of goods and services grew about 60 per cent. Between 1930 and 1968 the population grew by 63 per cent, but the consumption of crude petroleum increased by 300 per cent and that of natural gas by nearly 900 per cent.

"For the time being, Taeuber believes, the population growth rate is 'not a threat to very much of anything.' "

Further, President Nixon's National Goals Research Staff believes, "We have before us a set of decisions. One which appears not to be urgent is that of overall size of the population—even after the effects of a considerable amount of immigration are taken into account." At the present time immigration contributes about 20 percent to the rate of population growth in the United States.

WORLD SITUATION

Turning to the world situation . . . . obviously, the population has increased exponentially with time. If current birthrates are used to estimate future populations, the results are astronomical. But, as noted earlier, extrapolations are questionable. In this rapidly changing world, the factors that govern population growth, especially birth control, are changing with equal rapidity. This is pointed out by Donald J. Bogue, director of the Family Planning Center, University of Chicago, who says, "For more than a century, demographers have terrorized themselves, each other, and the public at large with the essential hopelessness, inevitability and morale-breaking pessimism of the 'population explosion' via exponential growth. Their prophecies have all been dependent upon one premise: 'If recent trends continue . . . .' It is an ancient statistical fallacy to perform extrapolations upon this premise when in fact the premise is invalid. It is the major point of this paper that recent trends have *not* continued, nor will they be likely to do so. Instead, there have been some new and recent developments that make it plausible to expect a much more rapid pace in fertility control."[9a]

Table 4 shows that there are many countries and areas in the world that are still sparsely populated. Australia and Canada actually need more people and encourage immigration. When one travels over the pampas of Argentina, the wheatlands of Canada, the rolling country-side of Australia, the great heartland of America, as I have done, he cannot help but be impressed by the open spaces that still exist. And I have been amazed at the open countryside in such lands as Thailand, Malaysia, India, Iran, Israel, and Western Europe. And even though there is little open countryside left in Japan, there are still many beautiful, secluded places where one can commune with nature.

Nevertheless, birth control will continue to spread in the developing countries, especially as new and more convenient contraceptive techniques are devised, because it is estimated that in these countries the number of live births per woman is 30 percent greater than the number desired.[10]

Without a doubt, the most critical factor in the developing countries is the food supply. Population growth rates have far exceeded rates of yield increase, whereas the reverse is true in developed countries. Overall, the rate of increase of food production in the world has about kept pace with the rate of increase of population. However, food needs will continue to rise from two main sources: increased population and increased per capita income leading to increased per capita consumption.

What about the future, then? According to Charles E. Kellogg, deputy administrator of the U.S. Soil Conservation Service and probably the world's leading authority on the soils of the world, the arable land of the world amounts to about 6,589 million acres. This is not quite twice the figure that the Food and Agricultural Organization of the United Nations gave in 1961 for the arable land in use. Later he revised this figure upwards.[11] Hence, there is no shortage of arable land at present, nor will there be for a long time. Much of this land is in developing countries in areas such as Africa and South America. As new technology develops, land that is thought now to be submarginal will be reclassified as arable. Dr. George Harrar, president of the Rockefeller Foundation, estimates that with present technology, food output could be doubled or trebled without bringing one additional acre into cultivation.[12]

Thus, without stretching the imagination, one can see how a combination of cultivating presently unused lands and applying modern technology could increase world food output about sixfold. Even this may be conservative. The new wheats developed in Mexico under the leadership of Norman Borlaug, recent Nobel Prize winner, have phenomenal potential. In using them, yields per acre have been trebled in Mexico and doubled in the United States and parts of India, Pakistan, and Turkey. It must be emphasized that these increases cannot be achieved without good fertilization and soil management. The new wheats are credited with breaking a yield barrier that has persisted for thirty years in India, a country that has more than a million new mouths to feed each month. And they have converted Pakistan into an exporter rather than an importer of wheat.

Patterned after the new wheat varieties, new varieties of rice have been developed by the International Rice Institute in the Philippines. Their yields are equally spectacular. The claim has been made by L. R. Brown of the Overseas

Development Council that "miracle rice is going to affect more people than any other technological development in history because, of the 3.5 billion people in the world, 1 billion eat rice." Because of new rice varieties, the Philippines and Pakistan became self-sufficient in rice in 1968, and India expects to grow all it needs by 1972. In fact, India's overall cereal crop is expanding more rapidly than population.

The most serious limiting factor in food production around the world is water. Think of the arid areas of North Africa, central Australia, the Middle East, China, and the great American Southwest. These arid areas could produce abundantly if water were available. Fortunately, man's ingenuity may take care of this problem. Alvin N. Weinberg has written on the desalinization of seawater as it relates to agriculture.[13] He believes that seawater can be desalted by using part of the energy generated in a nuclear-powered agro-industrial complex. Cost of desalting could easily fall to between 10 and 20 cents per 1,000 gallons, which is cheap enough to produce wheat at competitive prices. I have talked several times to Dr. Perry R. Stout (director of the Kearney Foundation of Soil Science, University of California at Davis), and he enthusiastically shares Weinberg's views. He has his own plan for such a complex in India. Of course, nuclear energy could also be used to pump the desalted water to where it is needed. Thus, it is not impossible that water could cease to be a limiting factor in the future and that the arid areas of the world could be made to "blossom as the rose."

If the agriculture of the world could be as efficient as that in Israel, there would be no need to worry about food for many generations. Recently I had the opportunity to travel over most of Israel in company with Israeli soil scientists. They showed me many facets of their agriculture. They are understandably proud of their achievements. In the northern part of Israel, in the hills west of the Sea of Galilee, I saw orchards that were made by leveling off the tops of hills with bulldozers. Bordering the orchards were huge rocks that had been moved aside. The soil that was left was still mostly rocks, but trees were growing and producing. On the shores of the Dead Sea I saw a hydroponics operation. There they were farming "the climate." They could produce such products as peppers and tomatoes earlier than elsewhere. Consequently, they received a premium for what they produced. Down near the Red Sea I saw fields being irrigated with irrigation water that was too salty by most standards. Still the crops were growing and being harvested. Israeli farmers now produce 75 percent (by value) of the country's food. Even surpluses exist for some agricultural products. This kind of production would not normally be expected from such an arid land.

That the world's food needs can be met in the future is attested by many of those engaged in agriculture. Professor V. W. Ruttan of the University of Minnesota, after reviewing three recent books on world food production, said, "Clearly the technical and economic capacity exists, or can be created by investment in agricultural experimentation capacity and in the industrial capacity, to produce the essential chemical and mechanical inputs, to meet world food requirements for the foreseeable future."[14] R. T. F. King, of the University of Cambridge, agrees. He says, "It appears to be technically feasible to feed the growing population of the world, but, as noted, it may cost more per unit of output to do so, and so food prices may rise."[15]

Recently I talked to Dr. R. C. Pickett, a colleague of mine in the Agronomy Department at Purdue University. He has traveled to nearly every country in the world, usually more than once, in search of sorghum varieties that might be used in plant breeding programs aimed at relieving the world's food needs. He has as much firsthand knowledge of agricultural conditions throughout the world as any man I know. It was gratifying to hear him say that, with the proper use of current technology and the land available to them, most of the countries of the world, including the developing ones, could be self-sufficient in food. Other references could be given. Nevertheless, those already cited should suffice to indicate that the problem of feeding the world is not insoluble.

I would not want to leave the impression that agricultural scientists are not concerned about the world's food problem. Also, it must honestly be admitted that not all agricultural scientists are as optimistic as those whom I have cited. The reason for this is not hard to see. *If* the world's population continues to

Table 5. Time Required for the Population to Double			
Annual Growth Rate (%)	Doubling Time (years)[1]	Annual Growth Rate (%)	Doubling Time (years)[1]
0.4	173	1.8	38
0.6	116	2.0	35
0.8	87	2.2	31
1.0	69	2.4	29
1.2	58	2.6	27
1.4	50	2.8	25
1.6	43	3.0	23

[1]To the nearest year.

increase at the present rate of 1.9 percent per year (Table 4), it will double every thirty-five to thirty-eight years (Table 5). The difficulty is compounded by the fact that the highest rates of growth are in the developing countries. In some of these countries 40 to 45 percent of the people are under fifteen years of age. Yet these are the countries where the prospect of increased agricultural production is the poorest. Therefore, it is not uncommon for agricultural scientists to recommend that the growth of the world's population be curtailed. But, in general, they see no need for the drastic measures referred to earlier. Unlike those who are less well informed, they don't demand emergency action.

As a matter of fact, it is difficult to predict what will happen in the future. As one agricultural scientist put it: "Beyond the end of this century we begin to pass into a science-fiction world in which neither the food that will be eaten nor the manner of producing it will necessarily be the same as today."[16] How much can we increase photosynthetic efficiency? Is there a way in which we can increase the amount of food the ocean can supply? What about synthetic foods made from petroleum and other natural resources? Can arctic regions and deserts be made productive? It is highly likely that other factors will become critical sooner than the food supply. . . .

Footnotes

1. Ansley J. Coale, *Science,* vol. 170 (1970), pp. 132-136.
2. See T. C. Jermann, *National Observer,* July 27, 1970.
3. R.F. Daly, *U.S. Department of Agriculture Yearbook,* 1970, pp. 87-92.
4. "Toward Balanced Growth: Quantity with Quality," Report of the National Goals Research Staff, Washington, D.C., July 4, 1970.
5. L.R. Brown, American Society of Agronomy Special Publication No. 6, 1965, pp. 3-22.
6. H.C. Wallich, *Newsweek,* June 29, 1970.
7. Jermann, op. cit.
8. A.M. Weinberg and R.P. Hammond, *American Scientist,* vol. 58 (1970), pp. 412-18.
9. L. Bumpass and C.F. Westoff, *Science,* vol. 169 (1970), pp. 1177-82.
9a. D.J. Beque, in *Alternatives for Balancing World Food Production Needs* (Iowa State University Press, 1967), pp. 72-85.
10. I.L. Bennett, *Food for Billions,* American Society of Agronomy Special Publication No. 11, 1968, pp. 1-16.
11. C.E. Kellog, *U.S. Department of Agriculture Yearbook,* 1964, pp. 57-69; *Alternatives for Balancing World Food Production Needs* (Iowa State University Press, 1967), pp. 98-111.
12. J.G. Harrar, *The Race Between Procreation and Food Production* (New York: The Rockefeller Foundation, 1965).

13. A.M. Weinberg, *Research with a Mission,* American Society of Agronomy
     Special Publications No. 14, 1969, pp. 1-14.
14. V.W. Ruttan, *Science,* vol. 168 (1970), pp. 690-91.
15. R.T.F. King, *Population and Food Supply* (Cambridge University Press,
     1969), pp. 28-46.
16. Ibid.

U.S. Population Growth: Would Slower Be Better?

Lawrence A. Mayer

The movement to curb population growth in the U.S. has come into prominence, curiously enough, at a time when the birth rate is close to its all-time low. The actual low in the U.S. birth rate came in 1968, at 17.5 per thousand. While the rate rose a bit to 17.7 last year—the first increase in more than a decade—it was still lower than at any point during the great depression of the Thirties. And though the number of births last year was up 2 percent to 3,570,000, that total was about 700,000 below the all-time peak reached in 1957.

The U.S., then, appears to have already moved in the direction that proponents of population stability advocate. But it's not at stability yet. Even at the recent reduced birth rates, the population has been growing 1 percent a year, and that is enough to double it in a single lifetime of seventy-two years. Moreover, birth rates are now bound to go higher, at least for some years to come. One important reason has to do with the changing numbers of women aged twenty to thirty-four, who account for about three-quarters of all births. This size of this group remained practically constant at about 18 million between 1955 and 1965, but from 1965 to 1970 it grew by three million, and in the next fifteen years it will increase ten million more. This wave of younger women is the result, of course, of the baby boom that followed World War II.

While the number of young women began to increase markedly in the years following 1965, the number of births did not. The women who had reached at least the age of twenty-five by around 1965 had borne most of their children by that time, and births to them naturally slowed down drastically thereafter. At the same time, women who were then just moving into the childbearing ages delayed having children (see "Why the U.S. Population *Isn't* Exploding," FORTUNE, April, 1967). This delay should partly be made up at later ages, however, and meanwhile the ranks of the twenty- to thirty-four-year-olds will increase rapidly. These two factors virtually guarantee that there will be a rise in births during the years directly ahead.

Reprinted from the June, 1970 issue of *Fortune Magazine* by special permission; © Time Inc.

How boomy this baby boom will turn out to be is a question that perplexes demographers. Those at the Census Bureau who made four alternative population projections in 1967 have already discarded the highest as virtually impossible (see chart, page 218). What's more, it has become clear that the second highest is improbable. Up to this moment, it is the lowest that is on target with a figure of 205 million for 1970*. At any rate Census will soon issue a new, lower set of projections.

In the present era of changing mores and social upheavals, it is even more difficult than usual to forecast the probable course of U.S. population growth. Just about everything known, however, suggests to Census demographers that a range of projections for the year 2000 should at the outside be no higher than 325 million (the old Census high was 361 million). Even the 300 million people still commonly said to be inevitable by 2000 are no longer inevitable at all.

SOME DISTANCE FROM ZERO

Population projections have to be built on many assumptions. One key assumption has to do with how large a family the average woman eventually will have. And nobody knows what that figure will be for the young women who will soon begin to bear children, or have recently begun. Surveys have shown that women expect what averages out as about 3.2 children. Demographers largely agree that at present it looks as if today's young women would have fewer children than that. But it would take a drop all the way down to an average of 2.1 children per woman (a bit more than 2.2 per married woman) to bring population growth to a halt. The 2.1 figure is sometimes referred to as the "zero population growth" rate. Obviously it takes two children to replace a set of parents. The extra 0.1 compensates for the girls who die before maturity and takes account of the fact that fewer girls than boys are born. (The 2.1 figure ignores net immigration, which has been contributing 0.2 percent a year to U.S. population growth.)

An important clue to future family size is the total fertility rate. This is the combined rate at which, in any particular year, women of all reproductive ages bear children. The figure for 1969 suggested women were building families at a rate that, if sustained, would give them an average of about 2.5 children by the end of their childbearing careers. This rate is very close to that underlying the present Census low projection. But the total fertility rate at any point in time may be an unreliable indicator. For example, the rate hit 3.7 per woman in the late 1950's, a figure demographers rightly suspected was too high to last. Many experts think the present 2.5 is too low to last.

---

*If this year's Census picked up the number of people thought to have been missed in the Census of 1960, the official figure for 1970 will finally be reported as about 210 million.

Donald J. Bogue, a demographer at the University of Chicago, argues that the present fertility rate is *not* misleading. The rise in fertility that followed World War II, he believes, was merely a prolonged interruption of the decline in the U.S. birth rate that got started early in the nineteenth century. He thinks it quite significant that by 1968 white women were bearing children at the rate of only 2.37 per woman, 1.26 fewer than in 1957 and not so very far from the stability rate of 2.1. Childbearing by black women (who account for about 17 percent of all births) has come down by about the same proportion, and was at a rate of 3.2 per woman in 1968. Moreover, Bogue thinks the black rate may go below the white rate by the end of this century. He points out, for example, that the percentage of black women who bear five or more children has halved since 1957. Moreover, college-educated black women expect fewer children than college-educated white women expect.

Accordingly, Bogue sees comparatively moderate growth in the U.S. population by the year 2000. The low of about 280 million in the Census Bureau's 1967 projection is the top of Bogue's high range. Bogue's low goes down to 220 million.

THE BIG LITTLE DIFFERENCE

A view quite different from Bogue's is advanced by Arthur A. Campbell, a widely respected government demographer now at the National Institutes of Health. He believes that the total fertility rate is probably giving off a false signal. He takes the depression years, when all measures of births were extremely low, as his bench mark. At that time, women born in 1909 were in their peak childbearing years. By age twenty-six (in 1935) they had given birth to about 1.05 children on average, and they finally produced the smallest American families on record, 2.23 children. By contrast, when women born in 1943 were twenty-six years old (in 1969), they had already averaged 1.57 children. It now looks as if these younger women would eventually have an average of close to three. Recent patterns suggest that 90 percent of today's young women will have at least one child; in contrast, nearly 25 percent of the women born in 1909 never had any children at all.

In short, Campbell believes that much of the recent decline in birth rates reflects a delay in childbearing by young women. And even though such delays tend to reduce the eventual size of families ("Later means less," demographers say), he still thinks current reproductive behavior is consistent with an average of 2.8 children per woman rather than 2.5. This seemingly insignificant difference has large implications. If sustained over thirty years to 2000, the higher figure would mean 25 million more Americans.

As surer means of birth control come into use, it becomes more important for demographers to know how many children people really want. One kind of

U.S. population
by age: 1970

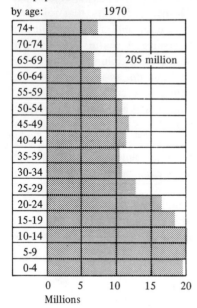

Variations on the Population Profile

These charts illustrate how changes in rates of population growth affect not only total numbers but also the age structure. The present profile reflects both the marked rise in births beginning in the 1940's and the leveling out and decline in births since 1957. If women continue to have families of present (or recent) size, the population will grow 50 percent by the year 2000 and will shift to a still younger age structure. But if family size declines to the "zero population growth" level by 1975, there will be similar numbers of people in all age brackets up to about fifty by the year 2000. (Data from Stephen Enke of G.E.-TEMOP.)

2000—if present family-size pattern continues

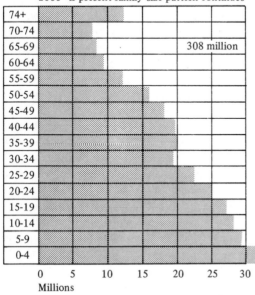

2000—"Zero population growth"

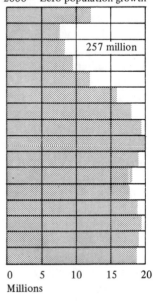

information bearing on this question is what proportion of births represents unwanted children. In a recent paper, Professors Larry Bumpass of Wisconsin and Charles F. Westoff of Princeton maintain that 16 percent of the births to women who were nearing the end of their childbearing years in 1965—when the last national fertility survey was taken—were unwanted. They conclude that these women, on average, would have had only 2.5 children if they had been able to exercise perfect control over their fertility.

This is astounding, since whenever surveys have directly asked women how many children they wanted or expected, the average has always come out a little over three. Bumpass and Westoff, however, went back over the 1965 questionnaires to ascertain what parents said about wanting *each successive child*. In this way the two demographers arrived at their 2.5 figure. And this result could well be conservative. It can be imagined that parents find it difficult to describe children who may literally be sitting in the adjoining room as "unwanted."

By extending their analysis to the entire population, Bumpass and Westoff conclude that in the 1960's one-fifth of all births were unwanted—meaning about 700,000 annually in the past few years. The extra births are more widely spread among social classes than might be supposed. The poor and near-poor, of course, contributed more than their proportionate share, *but more than half* of the unwanted children were born to parents who were not considered poor. (A family of four that had an income of at least $4,000 in 1964 was classified as "nonpoor.")

The implications of these findings are quite far reaching. If the number of children that couples really want average 2.5 rather than three or so, it might not require very extensive social alterations to attain population stability, assuming the availability of perfect contraception.

THE "POPULLUTION" PROBLEM

A sense that population growth is becoming a burden rather than a boon has taken hold in the U.S. with surprising swiftness. Last July, only a year after President Johnson's restrained advocacy of family planning and his hesitant mention of "population change," President Nixon spoke out forthrightly about the "pressing problems" associated with population growth. In keeping with Mr. Nixon's request, Congress has established a Commission on Population Growth and the American Future.

All the attention to population has arisen from several interwoven concerns having to do with crowding, pollution, and deterioration of the environment. The U.S. is confronting a "popullution" problem, observes S. Fred Singer, Deputy Assistant Secretary of the Interior and director of that department's research on environmental quality. Also, it is disturbing to some that the U.S. is chewing up a disproportionate share of the earth's limited stock of natural resources.

Population growth, of course, is not the only villain in these matters. Under present arrangements, the nation's productive system provides high levels of consumption but also throws off inordinate amounts of pollution, waste, and discomfort. The uneven distribution of the population also affects the quality of life.

It is often said that the U.S. doesn't really have a population problem, because there are only fifty-five people per square mile (sixty-five excluding Alaska). Density in some European countries runs more than ten times as high. But the over-all density figure for the U.S. is misleading, because two-thirds of the population lives in metropolitan areas, where density is much greater. And nearly half of the people in metropolitan areas live in central cities, where the density averages around 7,000 per square mile (and a lot higher than that in city cores). It is true that these urban areas are becoming decentralized, but the continuing helter-skelter growth of suburbs is causing new problems of traffic, water supply, and pollution.

If the U.S. rationally altered the distribution of people, it is often contended, there would be no reason for concern about the size of the population. This is more easily proposed than done. Schemes to distribute the population differently are up against what appears to be an iron law of urbanization: in a technologically advancing society the bigger cities tend to grow in perpetuity. Public authorities have tried over the years to halt the growth of London, Paris, Tokyo, and Moscow. None has succeeded, not even the authoritarian government of the U.S.S.R.

Another often-mentioned possibility is to build new towns. Britain has carried out the largest endeavors along this line, having started twenty-seven new towns—new cities, really—since 1946. But they contain only about 1 percent of the total population. Most observers give Britain's new towns at least passing marks, in large part because they have preserved a lot of open space, especially around London. However, the towns have failed to improve conditions within London; the inferior housing that was evacuated filled up again with newcomers.

Only a few communities that really qualify as new towns have been built in the U.S., and those few are not very populous. Recently the federal government gave its first real support to a new town in more than thirty years by issuing a loan guarantee to Jonathan, about twenty miles from Minneapolis. The location of Jonathan supports those who contend that new towns can succeed only within the ambit of established cities. If that is true, then although new towns prevent haphazard development, they don't really do much redistributing. A number of experts think some redistribution could be accomplished if new towns were built around existing ones and used facilities already in place. They have in mind cities in the Middle West that could stand revival—cities with

20,000 to 40,000 people that have stopped growing or are losing population.

One way to try to get new cities built is for the federal government to grant tax incentives to business, an approach that a number of studies and some bills in Congress advocate. Other measures that Washington or local governments could try include selective placement of procurement contracts, provision of inter-area job information, and special channeling of assistance to home building. This spring the Nixon Administration was considering several alternative approaches to a new-town program.

ROMANTIC NONSENSE

Many economists take a quite different approach to the problems of population distribution. Attempts to use subsidies and special assistance to get people and companies to relocate in less crowded parts of the country are "romantic nonsense," according to Dick Netzer, an urban-economics specialist at New York University. Of the many underlying reasons, perhaps the most important is that the key decisions about location are ordinarily not made by individuals seeking amenities, but by business organizations that cluster together in places they find economically advantageous.

The sensible way to change present patterns of distribution, Netzer and other economists maintain, is to make organizations and individuals pay the full costs of their activities. The argument is that if business, for one, was forced to pay for all the pollution, waste disposal, and traffic congestion resulting from its activities, and for all the benefits it gets from airports, highways, and other public facilities, the distribution of industry and people would be a lot different and the condition of the environment a lot better. In other words, the costs of producing and distributing goods and services should reflect the "externalities." The additional costs would, in many cases, be passed on to consumers. (See "The Economics of Environmental Quality," FORTUNE, February.)

Another way to reduce adverse effects of population growth on the environment is to reduce standards of consumption. It has been calculated that an attempt to get pollution in 1965 back to the levels of 1940 would have required reductions of 50 percent in the number of cars on the road, 50 percent in consumption of paper, 70 percent in generation of electric power, and 87 percent in the use of nitrogen fertilizer.

Still another set of troublesome questions connected with population has to do with the future adequacy of resources. The answers are by no means certain, though judging by the past alone there is nothing much to worry about. Important new materials such as petroleum and aluminum have been brought into use in the past century, and others, such as synthetic fibers and plastics, have emerged from laboratories. Additional reserves of minerals and fuels keep coming along. Better conservation methods have also added to supplies, as in the case of lumber. And improved technology has in some instances played an important role in holding down the consumption of materials. In 1968, electric utilities burned 480 million tons of fuel, measured in coal equivalents; Hans H. Landsberg of Resources for the Future calculates that 740 million tons would have been burned if the technology of 1940 had still been in use.

In principle there are only four real resources: the earth and its minerals, air, water, and fossil fuels. The first three can be constantly repurified or recycled in one way or another, maintains Roger Revelle of Harvard. But the fossil fuels—coal and petroleum—are irrecoverable once consumed, and are bound to run out within a few hundred years. However, most energy experts expect that, before the present century is over, breeder reactors to supply energy will be available, and some believe that controlled fusion will also prove feasible.

The world, of course, is a long way from ideal utilization and recycling of materials. Moreover, if one extrapolates demand on the assumption that most or all countries will become industrially advanced, then it is possible to arrive at enormously large estimates of future global requirements for resources. Changes in technology and patterns of resource use will temper these requirements, but even so, demand for materials will certainly rise far above present levels.

The U.S. is already a large user and importer of a long string of raw materials from antimony to zinc. With only 6 percent of the world's population, the U.S. gobbles up about one-third of the world's materials. At present the high U.S. rate of imports helps provide underdeveloped countries with badly needed foreign exchange, but as they achieve a high degree of industrialization they may ration their exports of resources.

AN EVENTUAL HALT

It seems feasible, in theory at least, to mitigate problems arising from the distribution of population, environmental pollution, and scarcity of resources by altering government regulations, taxes, and subsidies, re-allocating costs, and adopting different technologies and life styles. But such measures, even if society is willing to accept the costs, will not enable the U.S. to postpone indefinitely facing questions about population growth. Eventually, growth will have to come to a halt. Though no one can formulate them with any precision, there must be limits to how many people the earth, or any nation, can hold. Accordingly, it might be wise to begin thinking now about ways to stabilize the population. If society waits until limitation becomes a matter of desperate urgency, it may be too late for humane, noncoercive policies, and in any event the quality of life will have been severely and perhaps irreparably impaired.

The economic and social consequences of population stability merit a great deal more research and thought than they have received. Still, it is possible now to foresee some of the effects. Whether the effects seem beneficial or not depends to some extent on individual values and tastes; at any rate, a lot of things would be different.

It was once believed by businessmen and by many economists that population growth was necessary to sustain national prosperity. Nowadays hardly any economist would argue in favor of that view. Despite a widely held assumption to the contrary, big business seems to have swung around too. A FORTUNE-Yankelovich survey of chief executives of the 500 largest corporations (February) showed that almost eight in ten favor some sort of effort that would curb further population growth.

The size of the gross national product would be smaller with population stability than with continued growth. More women would presumably go to work if there were fewer children, but once employment of women reached a ceiling there would be no further growth in the labor force. From then on the economy could grow only as fast as the average output per worker. This means that if productivity is still rising at 3 percent or so a year with the population stabilized, the economy's potential rate of growth would be 3 percent a year rather than the present rate of more than 4 percent.

THE U.S. APPETITE FOR RESOURCES

U.S. Consumption as Percent of World Production

NATURAL GAS	67%	GYPSUM	29%
SILVER	58	MERCURY	28
MOLYBDENUM	50	CHROMIUM	28
SULPHUR	48	ANTIMONY	27
MAGNESIUM	43	ZINC	27
COBALT	41	CRUDE PETROLEUM	26
LEAD	37	TIN	26
PLATINUM	35	NICKEL	25
BAUXITE	30	COAL	21
COPPER	29	IRON ORE	21

The average standard of living is nevertheless likely to be higher with population stability. When population is rising, some proportion of national product must go to provide consumer goods and services and social overhead for additional people. With stability, the U.S. could use the freed resources to increase both private and public investment per capita. Because each member of the labor force would then be working with a larger or more advanced stock of capital, there would be more output and income *per worker*. And since workers would, on average, belong to smaller families, income *per person* would rise even faster. The income position of young families—with fewer children living at home than their counterparts of today—would benefit the most. It thus turns out that businessmen are confronted with a trade-off: a growing population would mean larger markets, and a stationary population would mean richer markets.

Markets would also be affected by the changed age composition of the population. By the year 2000, as the chart on page 218 shows, a population moving toward stability would have roughly the same number of people of each age up to about fifty. Several decades later, with population growth actually zero, all age groups except the very old would be approximately the same size. On the particular assumptions used to construct that chart, people under twenty-five would constitute one-third of the population compared to more than 45 percent at present, and the median age would be thirty-eight compared to twenty-eight. The market would thus be far more oriented toward older people and far less toward younger ones than is the case today. Apart from the different marketing strategies this implies, some industries would stand to gain, relatively, and others to lose.

With higher incomes and fewer children, young families could afford to spend more for travel, recreation, adult clothing, and home goods. The businesses that, on the whole, would presumably do worst are those with a kind of fundamental dependence on growth in numbers of people. Purveyors of goods and services for infants, producers of staple foods such as bread, sugar, and canned goods, bottlers of beer and soft drinks, construction, building-supply, and real-estate companies; and manufacturers of such tobacco products as are still being sold—all these could very well be stuck with relatively stagnant markets.

Population stability would also bring with it a somewhat less flexible economy, though it would not necessarily be less efficient. A growing population makes it easier to maintain opportunities for members of all occupations, and for business to make adjustments to changing tastes and technologies. Because markets grow faster, marginal investments are more likely to succeed and obsolete industries to hold on.

Stability is not likely to entail higher production costs. The U.S. market is already large enough to make it possible for most industries to enjoy maximum economies of scale, or it certainly will be by the time population growth levels out. At least one burden would grow, however. Social-security taxes and pension costs are bound to go up as stable population conditions are reached, because of the increase in the ratio of people receiving benefits to those paying.

WILL YOUTH BE DISSERVED?

Among the social benefits of population stability would be some reduction in poverty because there would be few large families. And smaller families would make for more education per child. That, in turn, implies a more highly skilled labor force and enhanced ability to innovate or to cope with advanced technology. The less the population grows, the less the need for increases in governmental expenditures in such areas as education, health, recreation, and water supply. Indeed, there would be less need for government regulation or intervention of many kinds. With relatively fewer young people around, there would presumably be less juvenile delinquency. With fewer drivers on the road, control of traffic would be less onerous. With fewer families looking for homes, there would be less pressure to alter the zoning of land.

Some people who have considered the matter maintain that population stability would bring some social disadvantages. Ansley Coale of Princeton has pointed out that when there are about as many older as younger people, the average age of those who run things will be greater, and advancement in business, in politics, or in any other form or organized activity will perforce be slower, a situation that will be frustrating to oncoming generations. Things might not work out quite that way, however: a relatively smaller demand for the services of young people would be partially balanced by a relatively smaller supply. In general, it may be misleading to project today's attitudes into tomorrow's world. A changed population structure would have many interacting consequences that might affect the morale and outlook of both young people and their elders in ways difficult to foresee. At any rate, it is not certain that youth would be served any less well in a stable population than it is now.

The most sweeping attack on population stability comes from the pen of Alfred Sauvy. This distinguished French demographer's textbook has finally been published in English (*General Theory of Population,* Basic Books), and may well play an important role in future debate about population. Sauvy presents a long catalogue of social, cultural, and economic ailments that France has experienced from early in the nineteenth century to the present, and he attributes them largely or exclusively to the virtual stagnation of the population during most of that time. The argument is long and rich, but cause and effect are scarcely ever conclusively demonstrated, and there is a noticeable absence of the statistical analysis one might expect. Sauvy's main explanation is that when population stops growing, society loses a sort of creative pressure that stimulates and adds healthy ferment to all of its aspects. This sort of generalization is perhaps more persuasive to French readers than to others, for concern over slow population growth is widespread in France and has been of long-standing concern to the government. Surely there are other reasons for difficulties that the French are bothered about. Coale likes to point out, for example, that just as the Industrial Revolution in England was getting under way, France, under Napoleon, was undertaking a series of ultimately unproductive military adventures.

ASSIGNED TO MOTHERHOOD

A society that wants to stabilize its population runs up against the puzzle of how to go about doing it. One difficulty is that little is known in any systematic way about the psychological and social motivations that impel people to become parents or to have large families. For example, to what degree are decisions to have children consciously arrived at and to what degree are they subconscious? Knowledge about such matters may be an important prerequisite for devising a population policy that would work.

Of course, if Bogue is correct that the U.S. is already moving toward a halt in population growth, there isn't any puzzle to solve. Or if Bumpass and Westoff are correct that the number of children women really want averages out to around 2.5, then perhaps a reasonably uncontroversial program might be able to reduce that number to 2.1. Such a program would include an education campaign about the long-run consequences of continued population growth; a system for making means of contraception available to all women; elimination of obstacles to abortion; and greatly intensified research efforts to discover more reliable and acceptable contraceptive methods. (At the moment, research is under way on some three dozen or so.) These steps would amount to a broadening and intensification of present family planning. Complete freedom of choice would be left to the individual.

But suppose Bumpass and Westoff are wrong, and people really still want three children? Then intensified family planning, though helpful, would be insufficient. Family planning in the U.S. has traditionally been put forward as a way of widening individual options, not of implementing a population policy. Some claim that family planning is incapable of fulfilling the latter role. The heart of the argument is that what demographers call "pro-natalist" influences are far too strong and deeply embedded to be counteracted solely by voluntary family planning.

Government tax and subsidy policies are at least implicitly pro-natalist. The examples that come to mind most easily are tax exemptions for children and, because of the split-income provision, higher tax rates for single than for married people. FHA and VA assistance to buyers of single-family homes has done a great deal to encourage the growth of all those child-centered suburbs. In many ways, customs and social arrangements operate to favor motherhood—a situation that some women are now vigorously protesting. Many people who advocate smaller families maintain that childbearing cannot be reduced substantially until women have real and satisfying alternatives to motherhood as a primary role. Perhaps nothing would do more to ensure the prevalence of small families than widespread success for the "women's liberation movement."

It will, of course, be somewhat easier to make a go of any limitationist policy once biologists learn just how to predetermine the sex of a child. In the U.S., as well as in other countries, many couples with one or more daughters decide to have additional children in the hope of having a son. However, if choosing the sex of children were to bring an appreciable change in the ratio of male to female births, that would not only enormously complicate population policy, but would also have other far-reaching social consequences.

A PROBLEM NEVER FACED BEFORE

There is some question whether a government can deliberately curtail a nation's population growth. Official approval apparently contributed to the postwar decline in Japan's population growth, but otherwise there is not direct evidence that government policies work. And the indirect evidence is negative. Some countries have consciously tried *pro*-natalist policies—France for the past thirty years, Germany under Hitler, Italy under Mussolini—with little success.

A great many proposed methods, some of them quite fanciful, have been put forward. Bernard Berelson, president of the Population Council, has listed twenty-nine different proposals to limit population growth apart from family planning. (Some really apply only to underdeveloped countries.) They include adding temporary sterilants—as yet undevised—to water-supply systems; licensing childbearing through permits that could be bought and sold on the open market, raising the legal age of marriage, and, of course, changing the tax system. The difficulty is to devise programs that are both feasible and effective. Measures that rank high on ethics, such as educational campaigns, might not be very effective. Deliberate changes in social institutions might eventually work, but they could have unforeseen side effects and would be hard to bring about.

Everyone who thinks about these matters is groping for answers to a problem that no democratic society has squarely faced before. The root question is how to reconcile long-run collective interest in limiting the growth of population with the desires of those who want to have more than two children. Uncomfortable choices will be involved if at some point society decides that it is desirable to curtail freedom to reproduce in order to preserve other freedoms or to preserve valued amenities.

Until recently almost all Americans took it for granted that the right to have as many children as one wants should not be abridged in any way. The number of people who openly disagree is a lot larger now than it was a few years ago, as is evidenced by the sudden emergence of the Zero Population Growth movement. The right to have children is not absolute, argues Judith Blake Davis, chairman of the department of demography at the University of California. She points out that much of the cost of the satisfaction enjoyed by families with many children is willy-nilly subsidized by others who must pay for the additional schooling and public services. The freedom to have children, she says, does not exist in a vacuum but in a context where the tax laws, the status of women, and various other social arrangements have a pronatalist bias.

SYMBOLIC COMMITMENT

It seems obvious that any population policy would have to meet certain ethical criteria. It should permit a maximum of individual freedom and diversity. It should not in any way impair the welfare of "extra" children. Also, it should not be used to practice selective coercion against any special group within the population.

The history and ways of Americans suggest that the fiscal system, which is impersonal and has long been used to accomplish social and economic ends, would come into play early in any effort to limit population growth. For example, there might be some form of bonus for not having more than a specified number of children. Or various kinds of tax disincentives might be enacted.

A proposal along these lines has been introduced in Congress by Senator Robert Packwood of Oregon. The bill would take effect in 1973 and would provide exemptions of $750 each for a family's first two children and none for any subsequent children. (Those born before the effective date of the act would not fall under this limitation, nor would adopted children.) Under tax provisions that were enacted last year and will take full effect in 1973, a family of four will get exemptions of $3,000 and a standard deduction of at least $1,000, so families below the poverty line won't be paying federal taxes anyway. The Packwood bill would therefore have no impact on large families among the poor. Nor would it have much impact on the well-to-do. The effect on people in middle-income brackets is uncertain, and Packwood, among others, suspects it wouldn't be great. "I don't regard a tax incentive per se as a key to population stabilization," he declares. "The important thing is that a tax-incentive bill, if passed, is a government commitment to make an effort to achieve stabilization. It would be symbolic."

Whatever the time or the circumstance, any policy of deliberately limiting population growth should be suffused with respect for the quality of individual life. This view was well expressed by Catherine S. Chilman, dean of the faculty at Hood College, in a paper recently presented at the New York Academy of Sciences. "We must care as a society," she said, "about the fulfillment and

well-being of individuals as whole people, not just as potential reproducers . . .
While a humane population policy would recognize the need to motivate people
to have no or very few children, it would lead from a social and psychological
base rather than one that is exclusively material and technological. It would
emphasize that there are many ways of being a respected, successful person
other than having a large family; that there are many benefits, other than
economic ones, alone, to be gained from controlling family size. It would build
on and enhance the human need to love, cherish, nurture, and protect."

VII. UNDERSTANDING

ENVIRONMENTAL EDUCATION

Environmental Education

When it began to dawn on people that the environment was worsening, that blight was creeping across our land, that the air was polluted and the waters running with waste, one of the first questioning glances was toward education. Our educational systems were caught off guard by the decline in environmental quality. They were no more ready to cope with the decay than any other part of society. Now in the face of the challenge the systems must be broadened to include new perceptions of environmental education.

What do we mean by "environmental education"? Nobody is certain. It has never been adequately defined. Education at least should help the student understand how the natural world works, not just its parts, but the relationships of one to another. He must appreciate not only man's dependence on and contribution to ecosystems, but the ways and degrees by which modern man alters them. As history cannot be adequately seen just as a series of acts, dates, battles, and names, but as the fabric of our past in relationship to our present, so environment cannot be seen but as a web of relationships.

This need not necessarily mean that ecology should replace any particular course of study or that education should be devoted entirely to ecology. But it does mean that there is a need for interdisciplinary education to cope with the interrelated nature of the environment. It is clear that man does not know enough about the environment around him and what he is doing to it. He has been a sorcerer's apprentice. He has loosed forces he only partly understands and can only partly cope with. It is not enough that experts know—and even they know precious little—but it is mandatory that the people who must live in the environment learn more about the forces that now move in sometimes dangerous ways upon it. Environmental education therefore is a key to making this a livable world.

That means, at the minimum, a fuller understanding of how the natural world works and how man is changing it. A better idea of how our economic systems and political institutions influence the choices that set off chain

Reprinted from *Environmental Quality,* The First Annual Report of the Council of Environmental Quality, Transmitted to the Congress, August 1970.

reactions wthin our environment, and a shift in personal values to make us willing to pay the price of controlling pollution, will both be necessary.

The Council is not ready yet to suggest how these needs must be woven into America's educational system. The picture is beset with too many conflicting, but legitimate, positions. They should be thoroughly debated.

Environmental education is not only "conservation education." Nor is it only the sum of the antipollution concerns that have recently captured public imagination. An "environmentally literate" individual is one who understands that he is part of a system composed of people, culture, and his physical and natural surroundings. He knows that man's acts can change his relationships to this system. He appreciates the human ability in some degree to control, preserve, and destroy the environment. He accepts responsibility for the condition of his environment. But that does not mean that he knows what to do about it.

A mere scientific study of earth's life support systems is inadequate. Environmental decisions are also based on economic and political factors, social pressures, and cultural values. Many Americans live most of their lives in cities. So it is essential that environmental education be relevant to them. That means that it must stress social and behavioral sciences. It should deal with what the student's environment is and might be. More colleges must begin to weave environmental content into science, technology, law, government, and education courses. And for the long run, perhaps more important than any of these actions, pre-school, elementary, and secondary school students must be exposed to environmental learning. That exposure involves curriculum development, teacher training, and organizational reform of a type and on a scale that do not now exist.

Pollution: The Challenge of Environmental Education

J. Alan Wagar

I am not an environmental educator. Rather I am a researcher concerned, among other things, with studying the effectiveness of communicating environmental information and concepts to the public. As such, I am an analyst who stands somewhat off to the side and examines what the problems are, how current efforts are working, what seems to be needed, and how improvements might be made.

From my slightly detached point of view, I conclude that we face an environmental crisis and that the challenge of environmental education is no less than that of preventing disaster for the human race.

Our environmental crisis comes from an arrested mentality that still assumes the environment can absorb any insult we can hurl at it. But along with this caveman mentality we have a modern technology and a command of energy that permit us to commit environmental errors that may not be reversible.

For example, two-thirds of the world is already hungry, but as a species we are reproducing as if the earth had no limit. The land that must support these populations has often been abused beyond repair. We are dumping such poisons as lead, asbestos, radioactive materials, and pesticides into the environment. Perhaps of greater importance, we are adding carbon dioxide and particulate matter to the atmosphere in great quantities. The increased carbon dioxide could conceivably cause the earth to warm enough to melt the ice caps and thereby flood most of the world's major cities. Or, the particles in the air might block out so much of the sun's heat that the earth could experience another ice age.

Some may think I am too pessimistic: After all, they could reason, despite the doomsday predictions over the centuries, man has survived all of his problems so far. Furthermore, it is his great skill in problem solving that has made man the dominant species on earth—a species that now numbers more than three-and-a-half billion and poses a major threat to any species that gets in his way.

Although contemporary problems are enormous, a host of specialists are

Reprinted by permission from *Today's Education* . *NEA Journal,* December 1970, pp. 15-18.

waiting to save us with schemes of many kinds. In view of all this talent, what is so important about environmental education?

In its simplest terms, environmental education is merely education for living effectively in an environmental situation that is turning out to be quite unlike what we have thought it to be. Our way of life is less and less appropriate to survival, and the task of correcting the situation is enormous, involving no less than a restructuring of some long-accepted attitudes in the American way of life. Essentially, we are talking about changing basic cultural values.

In trying to cope with the environmental crisis, we should avoid the witch-hunt approach of seeking "greedy corporations," "profiteering subdividers," "corrupt politicians," "misguided agencies," and "unscrupulous advertisers" upon whom to pile the blame. These people are not blameless and should not escape our scrutiny, but they are not so much the *causes* as they are *agents* for the rest of us. They can often claim—with some justice—that they are only practicing the good American virtues of progress, economic growth, free enterprise, and providing the public with an abundant life.

The blame comes home to roost. The causes, rather than being out there with "them," are right here with "us" and with some of our most cherished values.

Let me illustrate by reviewing some problems that spring from just four of our basic values: growth, laissez-faire, economic efficiency, and specialization.

First of all, we have an obsession with growth. This value made sense when a few settlers faced a nearly empty continent with vast spaces to be filled and rich resources to be tapped. In such an environment, an accelerating growth rate was feasible, even desirable.

But the earth is finite, and the end of growth is inevitable. Sooner or later, various limiting factors, such as lack of food or space and the diseases, parasites, and predators that flourish when a species is crowded, must slow down and eventually stop growth.

In all growing systems, there tends to be a slow start, a period of rapid growth, and finally a slowing and cessation of growth as various limiting factors are reached. When natural populations reach the levels at which limiting factors take effect, they can remain stable or they can become nearly extinct. (The latter occurred to the deer of the Kaibab Plateau, which become so numerous that they destroyed their food supply and then starved to death.)

Human populations, however, have a third alternative. Within limits, they can use technology to remove the limiting factors. This is exactly what has happened in the United States. Technology has so effectively removed the limiting factors encountered with population growth that we have come to believe in the possibility of an ever-expanding economy and ever-increasing growth. This belief, however, is complete nonsense in a finite world. If we avoid one limiting factor, another, perhaps more subtle, will take effect.

Currently, the limiting factors seem to be getting ahead of technology, and we are beginning to see that the effects of a growing economy include increasing smog, a vanishing countryside, the generation gap, death on our highways, crowded and substandard schools, growing restrictions on individual freedom, urban congestion, rising taxes, and a host of other problems.

At the same time that past growth has made future growth less and less desirable, it has also made some of our other values less and less effective. Our laissez-faire philosophy, for example, holds that the efforts of individuals to achieve their own self-interest will predictably lead to the common good. In pioneering times this assumption was often correct and workable because it provided the incentive for people to undertake the many tasks that needed doing.

But now there are many more of us, and we have growing access to mechanized energy that permits each of us to move about more and more. We occupy space directly by rushing about in automobiles, boats, and other conveyances and indirectly by requiring great factories, power plants, highways, transmission lines, and so on. Because we are all neighbors now, the decisions of one person affect many others. If one man decides his self-interest is best served by raising hogs or by installing a gravel crusher in his backyard or by gouging a mountainside or by filling an estuary, the effects on the neighbors are direct and highly disagreeable. As a friend of mine phrased it, "Not only are there more of us but each of us has bigger elbows."

Closely related to laissez-faire is the idea of economic efficiency. From the point of view of either the individual or of an organization, the cheapest way has usually been the best way. For example, in the interest of economy, waste products were normally just dumped into the water, into the air, or onto the land—regardless of their effect on others or on the total environment. In other words, dollar costs were the only costs recognized by the specific person or organization making a decision. The same reasoning has even been applied to public services. Many highway departments, for example, have been charged *by law* with the building of highways at the lowest dollar cost, even if somewhat greater dollar investments would do less damage to scenery, farmland, small communities, or fish and wildlife habitats.

Our passion for specilization grew as times became increasingly complex and the way to success lay in doing only one thing at a time. We purposely narrowed the view so that each specialist could delve deeply and solve problems of great difficulty in one small area of inquiry. But such specialization has more and more drawbacks. As John Muir pointed out long ago, you can't do just one thing at a time because there are always side effects.

When we lived in a very spacious environment and each of us had access to very limited amounts of energy, the side effects didn't gang up on us but were generally dissipated into harmlessness. People could rightly claim that "the solution to pollution is dilution." But now, when the side effects of our activities have become some of our major problems, we are stuck with experts who are so specialized that they are often unaware of side effects.

Many examples come to mind. The people who designed color TV were engineers, not medical scientists or geneticists, and they didn't know that some sets produced dangerous levels of X rays until after thousands of children had been exposed to them. Chemists, not ecologists, developed insecticides, and only after the damage was far advanced did they recognize that some insecticides were concentrated and passed along in biological food chains until they are now threatening eagles, falcons, ospreys, pelicans, and other species with extinction. Similarly, the specialists who developed automobiles weren't thinking of smog. The specialists who mechanized farming and thus cut down on the need for farm labor were not thinking of the consequent migration to the cities, which resulted in urban congestion with all its attendant problems.

The complexity of our society and technology is such that we must continue to rely on experts. But every expert must be sensitized to anticipate side effects and to recognize their growing importance. Part of every educated person's knowledge must be the idea that professional blindness to environmental consequences is no longer tolerable.

I have been saying that such values as growth, laissez-faire, economic efficiency, and specialization—values woven into the very fabric of our economic order—are also at the root of our fastest growing problems. If we don't modify these values, we face disaster.

On the other hand, disaster would be just as certain if we followed the suggestion of various campus radicals and summarily threw out the complex of values, technology, and organization that holds society together. Romantic as living without this "establishment" might be, we are far, far beyond the point of no return. To illustrate, it has been estimated that the entire earth would support only 10 million people at the hunting and gathering level of technology. North America alone might support two million. Currently, we have more than 100 times that many—vastly more people than can be maintained without all the technology and organization implied by the word *establishment*.

The upshot of all of this is that we don't have much room to maneuver. We must change our value system at a nearly explosive speed yet without destructive violence. In a society where government is by consent of the people, massive education offers us the only hope of avoiding disaster.

To meet this challenge, environmental education must involve far more than plant and animal identification for grade school kids. The crucial task is to provide every man, woman, and child in the nation with a deep ecological awareness of how all the things in our environment are interrelated.

Now that most of us live in cities, we are far removed from such realities as photosynthesis, soils, and food production. Many city people grow up thinking of milk as something technology provides to us in cartons. To them it has no relation to cows, grass, soils, sunshine, and acres of land. 'Yet these are the citizens who vote on crucial environmental issues. Environmental education has become essential for responsible citizenship.

Let's look at the needed changes in attitudes. Perhaps the starting point is to recognize that the earth is finite—a limited sphere. Having accepted this idea, we must recognize that unlimited growth is neither possible nor desirable and seek an approximately stable relationship with our environment. This will call for recycling as much of our material wealth as possible instead of using it and then discarding it. Currently, instead of a circular flow in which things are used repeatedly, we have a one-way flow—from resources through various processors and factories to consumers to junkyards. This one-way flow is depleting our resources and gorging our junkyards.

As part of a revised value system, we need to accept a new outlook on social accounting so that such things as clean air, safe streets, open spaces, and diversity are prized along with next year's automobiles and gold-plated plumbing fixtures. Often we will have to pay higher prices that cover *all* the costs of production, including repair of any damage done to the environment.

Within our present institutional framework, we can do this simply by changing the rules (and, of course, enforcing them), so that profit is taken out of doing the wrong things and incentive provided for doing the right things. A tax or charge on pollution and other environmental damage would create incentives for producers to find cheaper alternatives than dumping things into the environment and paying the charge. Such procedures would immediately bring technology and ingenuity to bear on problems in great need of solution.

There are sound scientific principles that determine the limits within which human populations, their environments, and their technologies can remain viable.

Attaining widespread understanding of the relationships between people and the environment is going to require massive education, involving all of the mass media. Fortunately, this is already taking place. Scarcely a day goes by without news coverage or a new magazine article on environmental problems.

Something deeper seems to be needed, however. All segments of the public need information that helps them see the nature of the problem and that helps them develop attitudes appropriate to the world as it is today.

To ask for change in deep-seated attitudes is stern medicine, and most people won't take it unless it is sugarcoated. Therefore, we need to place much of the burden on television. We should have prime-time programs that are dramatic and enjoyable enough to hold noncaptive audiences of all ages. Such programs could undoubtedly capitalize on the drama and even terror of what can happen if we don't change our ways. And, as I have mentioned, the villains must include our own inappropriate attitudes, not just convenient scapegoats.

To supplement and complement the mass media, the schools must introduce the basic concepts of ecology in the early grades as is already done in some places. Similar coverage must continue right on through college. This will require some tooling up, for at present there is a dearth of teachers equipped to do this. We also need to ask some searching questions about the content and effectiveness of the programs that do exist.

Since most of us cling to our basic attitudes unless we are under great stress, perhaps we won't change until the stress gets much greater. But by then we may have lost many valuable options.

What I am suggesting is that we have two basic choices. We can limit our growth and other impacts on the environment voluntarily, in which case the limiting factor is an *attraction* consisting of a life-style that provides space, abundance, freedom of many kinds, and a broad variety of alternative opportunities. Or, we can continue to grow and pollute and congest until stopped by *hardships*—limiting factors that are not of our own choosing. Instead of attractions, these will be constraints and repulsions, such as limited food, space, and resources; intense pollution; epidemics; greatly restricted alternatives on where we live and what we do; or a social pathology that paralyzes most of our efforts. Technology might deal with some of the problems, but only by imposing its own set of restrictions and problems.

As a species, we will probably survive, if we take no action, just as scattered and impoverished people survive on deserts that once supported rich agriculture and major civilizations. However, if Homo sapiens is truly a thinking being, we should seek much more than merely to survive environmental disaster. Attaining this "something more" is the challenge of environmental education.

Ecology — Heart of Our University Program

Edward W. Weidner

My article will describe how one institution of higher education—the University of Wisconsin-Green Bay—is responding to the environmental crisis by giving an environmental focus to its whole curriculum. We believe that if such a focus is to have a real impact on a national basis, many other schools at all levels must turn in the same direction. We do not suggest that other schools can or should copy directly what we are doing, for what each school does should be related to its own community and region and to the human and physical resources available to it.

The University of Wisconsin-Green Bay is a new institution. It was three years in the planning—from 1966 until 1969. We occupied our new main campus and launched our academic plan in the fall of 1969. Superficially, UWGB may appear to be like any other institution. We train chemists, biologists, physicists, and mathematicians. We train business administration specialists, elementary and secondary school teachers, artists, musicians, and actors. A student may select a foreign language, English, philosophy, or history. And all of the social sciences can be found in our course list.

The fact that much is familiar at UWGB is an important point to emphasize in an era that tends to emphasize the innovative and experimental. Every person who is going to be a responsible citizen of any modern society must master basic intellectual skills. In addition, many of our citizens need to master certain specialized skills. The question of critical social importance to which the UWGB academic plan particularly addresses itself is how each individual chooses to use the skills that he acquires.

As never before, our country and the world need citizens who are committed and dedicated to improving the lot of mankind. At UWGB, we are seeking to inculcate in all of our students a lifelong attitude of concern for the environment, its preservation and its improvement.

Our aim is to relate every part of our program to the ecological crisis. Whether it is teaching, research, or community outreach, the focus of the

Reprinted by permission from *Today's Education . NEA Journal,* December 1970, pp. 19-21.

university remains consistently that of helping student, professor, and community member to live in greater harmony with the environment and to *do* something constructive about the problems that beset it.

To carry out this mission, we must relate daily and directly to the people and to the other institutions and agencies of our community and region. Our students and faculty members must interact with the people of their community in identifying, investigating, and seeking solutions to the problems of their common environment. Conversely, we want the people of the community to think of the campus as a place where they and their ideas are welcome and where they can obtain resources and guidance. We have devised the label *communiversity* to describe this close reciprocal relationship and are doing everything we can to make UWGB a true communiversity.

Two fundamental ideas, then, determine our institutional direction: a focus on man and his environment, and the concept of the communiversity. In order to implement these ideas, we are forging an educational program that in a number of ways is different.

First, a true reciprocal relationship is developing between UWGB and the northeast Wisconsin region. Students and professors study, observe, and work in the community as well as in university classrooms. In turn, members of the community come into the classroom and interact with faculty and students. The teaching approach emphasizes problem solving and decision making in the context of relevance to environmental problems.

Second, teaching, research, and community outreach merge into a single intellectual function, as they must if we are to deal effectively with the pollution of a river, the decay of a downtown urban area, or any of the dozens of other environmental problems found in our region.

Third, a focus on ecology and communiversity requires extensive and frequent contacts between faculty and students outside the classroom as well as inside. It means a joint search for solutions to some of man's most urgent problems.

Fourth, students must take considerable initiative for their own learning. They must become skilled at sorting out their values clearly, identifying the major problems, and then getting enough information to develop programs of cooperative action to solve the problems.

Fifth, the primary focus of the curriculum is on environmental problems, rather than on individual disciplines and professional fields. UWGB recognizes and teaches the disciplines, but curriculum control is centered at an interdisciplinary level. Broadly defined environmental problems provide the focal points both for faculty organization and budgetary planning.

The UWGB student selects one of these environmental problem areas as the center of his intellectual interests. It may be a problem of the biophysical environment, such as environmental control in regard to air, water, land, natural resources, or environmental engineering. It may be a problem associated with social process, such as urban decay or regional planning. It may be one involving population dynamics, the ratio of available food to population, or the effect of environment on human development. It may deal with the matter of human identity and the many diverse aspects of human communication and action. If none of the formally defined problems satisfy the student, he may select an environmental problem of his own devising.

The environmental problem that the student chooses then becomes the central point of relevance for his program. He picks courses in the various disciplines and professional fields that contribute to thinking, problem solving, and decision making in connection with the particular environmental problem. Thus chemistry, art, secondary school teaching, psychology, or whatever subjects or activities make up his course program have new and exciting meaning for the student. They are means to a social end; they relate to one another, as well as to the environmental problem. The student learns to see the world outside the university as being fully as relevant to his learning objectives as the world of books, lectures, and discussions inside the university.

We think of UWGB as a new institution for a new age—the age of the environment. But a single institution, by itself, can have only very limited impact on the enormous problems that characterize this new age. Fortunately, during the past year, concern for the environment has become a popular theme throughout American society. Last Spring Earth Day captured the attention and the energies of millions of students at all levels of the educational system and also involved many adult citizens.

Many colleges and universities have added courses, institutes, centers, and seminars dealing with one or more aspects of the environmental crisis. The Congress and many state legislatures are beginning to piece together a new body of environmental law. Industry and government have begun to face up to the implications of their activities that pollute the environment.

This is all to the good, but it is only a first step. If we are to deal effectively over the long run with environmental problems, we must devise a coordinated network of institutional approaches. In many instances, of course, this will involve changing the orientation of existing institutions. Such changes are never easy and will require corresponding changes in the attitudes and goals of the people who make the institutions work.

The logical place to begin is in the educational system, particularly at the early levels where goal perception and attitude formation begin. We at UWGB are well aware of the need for developing a comprehensive plan for environmental education, starting at the preschool level and continuing through the elementary and secondary grades and on into all of the educational institutions above the secondary level.

Some time ago the Johnson Foundation of Racine, Wisconsin, became independently aware of this need. Recently UWGB and the Foundation agreed to pool some of their resources to begin practical study and field work for development of an environmental education curriculum for the K-12 grades. A three-year grant by the Foundation will cover a large portion of the salary of the full-time director of this project. We will need—and can get—substantial additional funding outside the regular university budget to carry out the project.

It is still too early to describe the project in any detail, but the current intention is to involve a number of public and private elementary and secondary schools in Wisconsin in the planning, preparation, and evaluation of curriculum materials. There will probably be teacher workshops, and certainly there will be an increasing interchange of ideas on this vitally important subject between the university and the school systems of the area.

With the support of a grant from the National Audubon Society, and in cooperation with the U.S. Office of Education and the Wisconsin Department of Public Instruction, UWGB is holding a national conference on environmental education on December 3-5. We expect this conference to generate guidelines and goals that can apply to our long-range environmental education project.

As one who has been intensively involved in the creation, staffing, and operation of a university that has man's environment as its single, strong focus, I am probably prejudiced. Nonetheless, let me express my profound conviction that every educator should be asking himself what he can do personally and professionally to help reverse the massive trend toward environmental degradation, a trend that threatens the entire life-support system of our planet.

What Secondary Schools Are Doing

☐ Pollution stands in danger of replacing the weather as a subject that elicits more talk than action.

But this is not true of a band of dedicated junior high students in San Bernardino, California, who work with the officially chartered Natural Beauty Program. These youngsters have added old-fashioned labor to their voices of protest about damage to the ecology.

Since 1958, successive members of the Conservation Club of Richardson Junior High, from which the Natural Beauty Program evolved, have collected tons of debris, planted scores of trees, and sponsored numerous activities that point up pollution problems to their elders as well as to their contemporaries.

In the fall of 1959, a committee of students from the Club visited the blackened hillsides that lay in the wake of a summer forest and brush fire that swept to the outskirts of the city. The loss of watershed, the potential for flooding, and the damage to the natural beauty of the area distressed the young people, and they decided to do something about it.

Working in cooperation with the U.S. Forest Service, the Club labored to repair the stricken area by planting more than 2,000 Jeffrey and Ponderosa pine seedlings; clearing stream beds; and building ponds, terraces, and check dams (constructed of the charred remains of trees), which prevent erosion from steep mountain terrain.

The project only whetted their appetites. The students became aware of the problems of pollution and blight. As disturbing to them as the actual problems was the public apathy that allowed these problems to exist.

The students began in-depth studies. In addition to visiting mountain, desert, and urban locations to see various problems, they went to sewage disposal and water reclamation plants, air-pollution-control and experiment stations, and similar installations.

Even while in transit to and from the points of interest in conservation studies, students saw defiling of the natural beauty of the area. Litter along the roadway worried them, and they classed it with air, water and noise pollution—

Reprinted by permission from *Today's Education*. *NEA Journal,* December 1970, pp. 22-24.

but with a difference: Here was a problem where they could take direct action. As students moved on in school and left the program, others came up to take their places, but not all of them left the program. Those who remain in the program as high school students form the program's board of directors.

In 1965, the daily press took note of a full-scale antilitter drive spearheaded by the Club, which had enlisted students from other schools and youth groups to their cause. It was then that the Club determined to organize the Natural Beauty Program of San Bernardino in order to recruit manpower to deal with environmental problems of the city and the area surrounding it.

By last year, the program had grown to encompass 2,500 young people from 22 different schools in the city school system along with members of the Boy Scouts, Girl Scouts, Camp Fire Girls, and others.

There were 36 separate antilitter drives last year, many of them school-neighborhood cleanups organized with the assistance of the Natural Beauty Program. Secondary school students and organized youth groups devoted a dozen Saturdays to these antilitter drives.

The program has a goal for the current school year of about 4,000 participants from the city schools, plus additional hundreds from the area's organized youth groups. Early fall fires in Southern California have created a real need for even greater dedication by the program's youngsters.

In another cooperative project with the U.S. Forest Service, the young people went to work to clean up the remains of an abandoned rubbish dump that had turned a canyon into an eyesore and threatened to pollute the underground water. During the year, 300 different youngsters contributed more than 800 man-hours of volunteer labor to reclamation of the old dumping grounds. They planted 650 trees and moved dirt and rock by hand to establish a parking lot in a strategic area for a scenic overlook.

Teachers and administrators close to the Program feel it helps to establish a stronger tie between teacher and student in addition to involving large numbers of youngsters in constructive citizenship. As one teacher put it: "When teachers put on their old clothes to help students clean the neighborhood of trash or kneel beside a boy or girl to plant a seedling, students find out their teachers are human."

—Gerald W. Stoops, *science teacher, Richardson Junior High School, San Bernardino, California.*

☐ Survival in the urban environment has become a major theme in my life-science program for students. Being located in the greater Detroit area gives students unlimited opportunity to conduct studies on environmental pollution. In the most successful studies, students carry on field investigations in the urban area that are ecological studies, *not* mere tours.

Student research teams generally divide into four groups, each responsible for conducting some aspect of the field investigation. Some students take photographs and movies of the area under study. At a later time, they use these visual records to determine if environmental-improvement programs are making any progress.

Other students record environmental data—for example, the climate, the nature of the topography, or the source of the pollution (steel plants, chemical plants, and the like). Still other students collect air, water, and soil samples. They also collect small animal and plant specimens, such as insects and weeds. And they record the general biological community in the area; noting and, if possible, identifying larger animals (birds, squirrels, rats) and plants.

From these field investigations, the biology students develop an ecological profile of the plant and animal communities that survive in a severely polluted urban environment. They correlate biogeographical data with specific sources of industrial pollution, and very interesting ecological maps of Detroit have resulted. Many biology students are conducting controlled experiments with the air, water, and soil samples collected during the field investigations. Some, for example, are growing plants in contaminated air and watering them with different industrial river samples. Some are making detailed ecological studies of aquatic and soil populations from samples collected in various regions of Detroit.

Recently, my biology students have undertaken several projects to study human ecology in the city and surrounding suburban areas. To them, the survival of human beings in a congested urban environment characterized by severe pollution has become a most pressing topic for discussion. Unfortunately, the more they discuss the topic, the more they become pessimistic about the future.

—Ronald Saltinski, *science instructor, grades 9 through 12, Robichaud High School, Dearborn Heights, Michigan.*

☐ The scientific demonstrations were dismantled, the free pamphlets were gone, the guests and speakers had departed, and yet the most important products of the April Environmental Symposium at Amity Regional High School—the newly acquired knowledge, the energy, and the commitment to redress the environmental balance—were there, ready to be guided. The aim of the symposium had been to increase awareness of the environmental crisis. The 1,000 participants had heard experts on all aspects of the problem; they had seen movies and scientific demonstrations.

Environmental happenings did not end with the symposium, however. The after-school Zero Population Growth environmental slide show provided an exciting assembly. The symposium awoke curiosity and concern and consequently triggered a number of activities that altered the spectator-sport image of the teach-in. Collecting litter around the high school as well as in the community and taking a bicycle inspection tour of New Haven began a list of student activities carried on after school.

During spring vacation a number of students and a teacher testified in an open hearing before Connecticut's Clean Air Commission, and a number of Amity students joined with high school and college students in the area participating in Earth Day events in New Haven.

Probably the most exciting and meaningful activity was the series of highly publicized mini teach-ins that 20 senior high students presented at the two junior high schools and several elementary schools in the community. With some additional research and some suggestions on creative presentation, the students took to the teaching field to transmit their new knowledge to eager ears. As one of the "student teachers" put it, "When the day was finished, I felt students had at least been exposed to and had grasped an understanding of the environmental problem. I am sure there was no monumental change in anyone's life, but if the teach-in challenged peoples' minds, then it was successful."

The symposium program has also influenced the Amity classroom in two important ways. First, it has given the classroom teacher the impetus to integrate various aspects of environmenatl problems into the curriculum. Second, it has resulted in an increased number of special research projects of a scientific as well as a socioeconomic nature. In general, each individual involved has a new aware-ness of his impact on environment.

This year a new student activity began: the Environmental Action Club. The Club's principal project is a program of recycling glass and metal. Members hope to educate residents of the community to separate waste that can be recycled from waste that can't. Money raised from the program will be used to develop an ongoing environmental education program, including future teach-ins, for students and community.

—Joseph Proffitt, *chairman, History Department;* Susanne Duffy, *history teacher;* James R. Bouchard, *biology teacher; and* Lawrence Schaefer, *chemistry teacher. Amity Regional Senior High School, Woodbridge, Connecticut.*

□   "A mourn-in for a marsh?" everyone asked in the early spring of 1969. Snow was still on the ground, and few people even knew what the word *ecology* meant, but the Thomas School's biology teacher, Joy Lee, was aware and determined to arouse her students and school to the crisis in their own backyard.

Located as it is on the shore of Long Island Sound, the Thomas School, a private girls' school, had long made use of the local marshes for biology field study. Aroused at the wanton filling and pollution of the local marshes by people who were unaware of the damage they were doing to the ecology of the area, Mrs. Lee discussed the situation with her students, who decided to do something about it.

Mrs. Lee asked my permission to start a public information campaign aimed at stopping the destruction of the marshes. Her plan was to begin school with an early morning breakfast for local politicians, state legislators, and conservationists. From there, the students would march to the local marshes wearing black armbands and carrying placards proclaiming a "mourn-in" for the dying marsh. I endorsed the proposal enthusiastically, and the movement was under way.

After the breakfast and the mourn-in, which received excellent newspaper coverage, the next steps came naturally. Thomas students set up an organization called PYE (Protect Your Environment). The students and their art director designed an emblem with blue and green triangles on a yellow disk to stand for clean air and water, green spaces and sunlight—elements necessary for the sustenance of life on earth. They made the new emblem available to the public as buttons and auto decals, which began to appear all over southern Connecticut, and eventually spread to other schools. Recently it appeared on the cover of *Scholastic Magazine.*

When PYE learned that a wetlands bill had long been bottled up in the Connecticut legislature, Mrs. Lee and her girls went to work. They prepared literature on the bill, went to the commuter stops at 6:00 A.M. and 7:00 P.M. to arouse voter interest, and bombarded the members of the legislature with letters, information, and PYE buttons. PYE girls went to Hartford with Mrs. Lee to appear at legislative committee hearings and they collared legislators in the halls of the state capitol. New York City's Channel 2 came to Thomas to do a two-minute spot for their evening news report and ended up giving 11 minutes of coverage to the PYE Club endeavors.

As a result of PYE's efforts, Connecticut Senate Bill 419 was reported out and was passed unanimously by the House and by voice vote in the Senate. On July 1, 1969, Governor Dempsey signed it into law. The most noteworthy provision of the bill is a moratorium on use of tidal areas until a survey can be made to determine what areas should be retained for the public domain and what areas can be made available for private use.

Since that time, PYE has become a nationally recognized movement of secondary school students and has helped more than 60 other schools from coast to coast establish their own PYE clubs. More than 90,000 PYE buttons and decals have been sold or distributed to schools, colleges, and interested adults.

PYE puts its weight behind members of Congress who are willing to work for legislation to save the environment. Plans are being laid to coordinate the efforts of the many PYE clubs to distribute information on voting records of various Congressmen, and to keep the ecological issue before the public and the politicians.

Last spring, PYE members went to Washington for conferences with a number of Congressmen and with Secretary of the Interior Hickel. Secretary Hickel and the Congressmen the PYE girls visited were friendly and receptive.

Of immediate interest to the PYE clubs of Connecticut is Senator Ribicoff's proposal concerning a tristate plan to clean up Long Island Sound. PYE clubs can help this kind of proposal through taking part in public-information programs.

Like all groups concerned with the growing environmental problem, PYE knows that the task ahead is seemingly insurmountable. Nevertheless, because of the public's growing awareness of the need to save such areas as the Rowayton Marshes, it is not dismayed by the gigantic cleanup that remains to be done.

—Arthur Harper, *headmaster, the Thomas School, Rowayton, Connecticut.*

We must . . . realize that we are going to have to rethink our standards of luxury and necessity. For instance, our use of electricity ought to be reconsidered.

The utilities fill our needs for electricity. We cannot, on the one hand, condemn utilities for making efforts to provide us with electricity, and then turn around and fill our homes with endless electrical gadgets. We demand from the utilities that they always supply us with enough electricity to run our electric toothbrushes, our electric knives, our electric blankets, our electric can openers, and all the other modern conveniences of our society. But we never stop to consider that because of our excessive electrical demands, the utilities must keep building and operating polluting power plants. The first step to help clean up pollution caused by overworked power companies is to reduce electrical demands that every home makes, and we should begin to seriously consider this fact now.

Charles H. Percy, *U.S. Senator from Illinois.*

What Elementary Schools Are Doing

☐ Last winter the sixth graders in Templeton Elementary School really grabbed hold of our science unit on land, air, and water pollution. In it we studied the causes, effects, and possible future solutions. We learned about pollution in our own community through a study done by a local environmental control agency.

Children started bringing in newspaper and magazine articles to report on, read, and discuss. Bulletin board displays flourished.

The facts we gathered about pollution alarmed the children. But it was in a language class that a group of them got excited about doing something themselves to tackle the problem. They decided to begin by educating the rest of the student body.

For the next few weeks, the children, working in interest groups, created puppet shows, skits, stories, slide presentations, picture and chalkboard demonstrations, and talks to give to the primary grades.

The kids didn't want to stop with this project and sought another more sophisticated one—an assembly on pollution to educate the intermediate grades. At this point, enthusiasm about the whole project caught on with all the sixth graders, and so the projects were easily carried out in science classes agian. Each class selected various media to illustrate the problem and solutions. At intervals throughout the assembly, students from one class gave short speeches that presented interesting and startling information about pollution. We gave this same program later on for our Parent Teacher Association.

During this time, volunteer groups of youngsters had been spending recesses picking up litter around our school grounds. The children initiated and carried out a final project entirely on their own. One Saturday a group of more than 20 drove around town in an old firetruck (obtained by the fireman father of one of the group) and picked up enough litter to fill more than 13 huge bags.

All these projects succeeded because our pupils were sufficiently concerned to do something about pollution above and beyond any school requirements.

Reprinted by permission from *Today's Education*. *NEA Journal,* December 1970, pp. 25-27.

Nell Cretsinger, *former sixth grade teacher, James Templeton Elementary School, Tigard, Oregon.*

☐ Since 1966, the Elyria, Ohio, City Schools have given considerable attention to the pollution problem and to expanding the curriculum to include a broader involvement with environmental education.

Last spring, 625 students in grades 3-6 from six Elyria elementary schools participated at a wooded campsite in a series of outdoor education studies that stressed nature sciences and art.

A second continuing program is built around the broad topic "Man, Art, and the Environment." Art teachers at all levels participate sometime during the year in planning with each art class a study unit derived from this topic.

Some activities have been limited to visual-descriptive interpretations of the environment, with paintings, posters, and graphic prints predominating. Some have pursued in-depth color studies based on pollution-casued environment changes, even reaching out to the long-range effects on adaptive, protective coloration in birds and insects.

Other activities have involved designing idealized two-and three-dimensional plans for better living spaces to accommodate man's city life without despoiling the environment.

As a result of cooperative planning, we have discovered that a close and natural working relationship can exist between the areas of art, social studies, and science and that this relationship needs to be capitalized on to coordinate studies involving man and his environment.

—Charles R. Rose, *supervisor of art education, Elyria, Ohio, City Schools.*

☐ "Gee, you can really tell the difference in the air now, can't you?" "Look at the exhaust from the car; bet the driver hasn't had his air pollution mechanisms checked." A group of elementary school students voiced comments such as these as they returned home after a three-day, camping-field trip that climaxed an experimental project in air-pollution-control education in the summer of 1969.

The project, which was carried on at the Institute of Child Studies at Newark State College, proved conclusively that elementary school students can become interested in and concerned about the control of air pollution.

Helped by a grant from the Kirby Foundation, the School of the Outdoors Foundation operated the project through the Institute, with College cooperation.

Every morning at 8:30, the "research team" (students who had just completed sixth grade) gathered at the "classroom" (a converted storage-workroom) for the day's explorations. With the exception of one half-hour swimming period and a long lunch-recreation period, we spent the day developing a resource unit that would enable students in middle school classes to learn about air-pollution control.

These were the project's guiding principles:

1. Since air pollution is an environmental problem, the outdoor education method should be a major part of the strategy.
2. Students should be involved in every phase of the project.
3. It should be a "doing" project, not just a listening or reading project.
4. Behavioral or instructional objectives offer a built-in means of partial evaluation.
5. A multidimensional strategy offers many opportunities for reinforcement.
6. A structure starting with basic concepts provides a logical basis for a program.
7. Inquiry and discovery should replace "cookbook" experimentation.

We started with concepts about air and its properties; moved on to weather and climate; and then into the next steps of correlating the effects of air pollution. Much of the learning experiences came about by *doing*. We had a homemade weather station and soon were making daily weather reports and forecasts. Before we finished, we added a pollution station. By this time, we had made devices for measuring some of the simpler pollution components. We measured particulate fallout in several places; practiced methods of making pollen counts; and, whenever possible, observed and studied the effect of the sun in producing other pollutants and in producing convection currents and winds.

In the "laboratory," we made and tried out various devices. For example, in "mini-greenhouses" made of flowerpots and plastic bags, we subjected growing plants to car exhaust fumes and obtained some dramatic results. All devices were made of readily available materials, in an ordinary workroom, and with tools and equipment anyone could get. Our basic supplies were tin cans, bottles, balloons, milk containers, wood from boxes, and an old vacuum cleaner, supplemented by aquarium tubing and a little laboratory glassware. One exception to the readily available category was a set of "detector tubes" for mine safety work, which we purchased. We developed an inexpensive pumping device. Since we were more concerned with awareness than with scientific measurements, the simple devices were adequate.

We did much work outdoors and took frequent field trips. We tested air at the seashore, on the highest mountain in the state, in a remote rural area, and in a city, as well as in our own suburban area. We visited pollution research centers to see what the professionals were doing. A three-day trip that climaxed our project gave us the opportunity to enjoy an unpolluted area and also provided a basis for contrast with polluted areas.

One set of experiments concerned the effect of air pollution on the human being. We made visibility tests, compared odors, and estimated lung capacity under different circumstances with a simple spirometer. The effect of air pollution on nerves and pulse rate and endurance as shown by simple activities fascinated the students.

Since one of our objectives was to present a multidimensional strategy, we also used films, filmstrips, discussion, occasional lectures, demonstrations, and all the reading matter we could find on the subject. At one point, our students taught lessons to a visiting group of retarded students with excellent results for both groups.

After the pilot project ended, an advisory committee of scientists and educators checked all the material thoroughly and put it in the form of a resource unit that others could try. Nine classes in the middle grades of five school systems thoughout the state tried out the program during the 1970 spring semester and provided very favorable feedback. The mid-Atlantic section of the Air Pollution Control Association is now considering the possibility of printing the unit and making it available for general use, free of cost, early in 1971.

We feel that this unit has much merit. We are sure that *every* school must include in *every* course of study information about air pollution and other environmental factors if the general public is to sustain the long-term effort needed to maintain a viable environment for man.

—Benton Cummings, *assistant professor of outdoor education, Newark State College, Union, New Jersey. Mr. Cummings taught biology and earth science at Newton (New Jersey) High School.*

☐ Two years ago—before the high pitch of concern over the "pollution crisis"—the small coastal community of Yarmouth, Maine, embarked on an exciting environmental education program for its 1,200 youngsters in grades K-12. The pilot program, entirely community-financed, was spearheaded by an energetic superintendent, a concerned and far-thinking school committee, and an industrial arts-science teacher, who served as coordinator after receiving special training during a year's leave of absence. The appeal of this first-year effort was contagious, and the second year found three neighboring school systems sharing the program.

The program focuses on the natural and man-made elements of the community—particularly its environmental problems and the role of citizens in helping to solve them. During the school year, as many as 50 citizen volunteers assist the coordinator and classroom teachers on outdoor field trips. This makes it possible to divide classes into small groups, enabling the leaders to reach each student as he explores the environment of his school (grades K-1), the neighborhood (grades 2-3), the community (grades 4-5), and the region (grade 6).

On the field trip, students get a firsthand look at the natural components of the study environment and at their interrelationships—land, water, air, plants, animals, and energy and its effects. But the exciting aspect of the program is that it encourages youngsters to investigate how we use these basic resources in our urban environment (through land and water development, structural design, transportation, ulitities, and recreation) and what environmental controls are needed to protect them. These themes are focal points for basic science and social studies concepts that students acquire through classroom presentations, field trips, and follow-up environmental improvement activities at all grade levels. The program is, therefore, interwoven throughout the curriculum in the school system.

Since the success of environmental education depends on going out beyond classroom walls, school site development is another major responsibility of the coordinator. Now well under way in Yarmouth is a model school site being developed for use as a teaching resource for environmental learning, a place where students can carry out environmental improvement or conservation activities, and a community outdoor recreational or nature center.

Still another area of work for the coordinator involves curriculum enrichment through special workshops, field trips, newsletters, book lists, and so on.

Today, the program is shared by four other communities—Falmouth, Freeport, Cumberland, and North Yarmouth—reaching over 6,000 students. What of the future? At least four more school districts in Maine have now agreed to establish and finance such model programs in their schools. In preparation for these programs (under a Title III ESEA grant), four teachers from these later school districts are now receiving a year of specialized training at the University of Michigan. How the state agency and university system of Maine can meet the needs of other schools is being explored.

And so a state that still has opportunities to protect its precious natural resources and plan their development is well on its way with a program that will support a statewide environmental policy.

—Dean B. Bennett, *director, Maine Environmental Education Project, Title III ESEA, and doctoral student in environmental education, University of Michigan. Mr. Bennett has taught at the elementary, secondary, and college levels.*

A Survey of School Environmental Programs

☐   In 1969-70, the NEA Research Division conducted a pilot study to find out what is being done at present to teach pupils in public schools about their environment. It did so under a contract funded by the National Park Service and administered by the American Association for Health, Physical Education, and Recreation (an NEA national affiliate) as part of Project Man's Environment, an environmental awareness effort undertaken by AAHPER. This study was the first attempt ever made to survey environmental education programs on a nationwide basis. It was designed as a survey of programs in environmental, outdoor, and conservation education in operation in public schools in 1969-70 and covered all grade levels from pre-kindergarten through adult education.

Because of the impracticality of covering all school systems in the country, the survey included only systems that enrolled 1,000 or more pupils; however, these school systems enroll 90 percent of all public school pupils in the United States.

To concentrate on reasonably extensive programs in environmental education, the survey was further limited to those systems that had the equivalent of at least a half-time staff person assigned to an environmental program. A return-postcard sent to superintendents of all school systems with enrollments of 1,000 or more identified systems with programs of this type. Those having such programs received a lengthy questionnaire asking them about various aspects of their programs. More than 700 systems (90 percent of those surveyed) returned completed questionnaires. The results of the survey apply to the environmental programs in operation in these 700 school systems.

The survey revealed considerable diversity in environmental education programs. Following are some of the major findings relating to programs in the survey as a whole:

• A majority of environmental education programs are entitled "Outdoor Education" and are intended either to give pupils a general acquaintance with the outdoors and nature or to provide them with a general awareness of man in relation to his environment.

Reprinted by permission from *Today's Education* . *NEA Journal,* December 1970, pp. 28-29.

- Programs are aimed chiefly at pupils in the upper elementary grades.
- A majority of programs operate either year-round or throughout the entire school year, but in most instances scheduling is limited to the regular week.
- The administration of most programs is centralized within the school system, but a considerable number of programs are administered on a decentralized basis.
- The great majority of programs combine classroom study with visits to sites outside the classroom. Almost all of these provide students with special preparation for their visits to sites and conduct follow-up activities afterwards. Discussions and reading in class, audiovisual presentations, and visits to the classroom by resource persons are all widely used as prior preparation for on-site experience. The most widely used types of follow-up activities involve oral reports and discussions; the examination, identification, and use of specimens gathered at the site; displays and exhibits; and written reports or essays. Films, slides, and transparencies, further reading, and art activities are also often used in follow-up of on-site experience.
- The areas of study included in the greatest number of programs are conservation, ecology, biology, insect study, geology, botany, general science, and weather study.
- The curriculum of programs is most often determined by an instructional team. In many cases, the teacher prepares field lessons for each trip, and student interests also influence curriculum planning.
- Most programs attempt to determine whether students' attitudes toward their environment have changed.
- Most programs that include students at the secondary level grant academic credit for work done in the program, but relatively few programs give grades.
- In a majority of programs, students visit places where they stay overnight. Most of these sites have cabins or bunkhouses, cooking and dining facilities, and an infirmary. The educational-recreational facilities most often found at such sites are indoor meeting rooms or classrooms, a display and exhibit center, a swimming area, and a crafts shop.
- Sites typically include forest or woodland, ponds or lakes, a recreation area, campgrounds, or a wildlife natural area.
- For a site that is used for day trips, 50 miles from the school district appears to be the maximum feasible distance; for overnight sites, 100 miles. Few school systems, however, actually impose restrictions on the distance students may travel to environmental study areas.
- Most programs use the services of regular school staff—classroom teachers and principals—with the assistance of a resource person. Part-time staffing of programs is more common than full-time staffing.
- The great majority of persons in charge of environmental education programs are academically well-qualified as educators, holding a master's degree

or higher, but few of them have had preservice training specifically in an area of environmental studies. However, most school systems with environmental programs provide in-service training opportunities for their staffs.

• Local sources of funds—chiefly, local boards of education—are of prime importance in financing environmental education programs.

• In addition to a basic need for increased financial support, a majority of programs in the survey acknowledge a need for assistance with instructional materials and in-service training guidelines in order to develop further.

The survey discovered three different types of environmental education programs related to the grade level of the students participating in them.

Some school systems, either because they are elementary systems or because of the design of their environmental programs, provide environmental education only to students at the elementary level. On the other hand, some systems offer environmental programs only in one or more of the junior or senior high grades. Still others offer environmental education at both elementary and secondary levels. The largest proportion of the programs included in this survey were of the combined type, including both elementary and secondary levels, but almost as many were restricted to the elementary grades, while only a small proportion were restricted to the junior-senior high grades.

These three types of programs are quite different from one another. Programs restricted to the elementary grades are usually one-year programs aimed at grade 6. They operate chiefly within the regular school week and often during only one season of the school year (fall or winter or spring). They are designed primarily to give pupils an appreciation of nature and an opportunity to enjoy the outdoors, and a large proportion of them are, in effect, camp programs in which student experiences are limited to a period of residence at a site.

On the other hand, programs restricted to the junior-senior high grades operate chiefly within the framework of the traditional academic curriculum. Most of them are two- or three-year programs, directed at the senior high grades, and the largest proportion operate through out the school year. They focus primarily on the technical and scientific aspects of environmental study. The largest proportion limit their activities to classroom work with selected field trips. Their students spend a greater amount of time in the classroom than do students in the other types of programs and usually receive both grades and academic credit for work.

Programs that include both elementary and secondary levels are more comprehensive than either of the other types. More than half include six or more elementary grades, and a large proportion include a similar number of secondary grades. Primarily middle grade programs, the great majority are directed at grades 4 through 8. They attempt a total approach to the study of man and his environment, covering many different aspects of the field. A large proportion of them operate year-round. Collectively, they include a wider range of areas of study, use a greater variety of sites, and employ more staff persons than do programs restricted to either the elementary or junior-senior high level.

This is only a preliminary survey of environmental education programs throughout the country. Much remains to be learned about efforts to increase environmental awareness through public education.

—*NEA Research Division.*

Environmental Education in the K-12 Span

LeVon Balzer

A widely accepted definition of environmental education is not available at the present time, in spite of the extensive emphasis upon the environment and environmental education. In addition, various terms are being used with a wide range of meanings. To clarify discussion in this paper, a brief discussion of some of these terms follows.

Nature study. This complex and diverse movement was initiated at the turn of the century by Liberty Hyde Bailey and associates at Cornell University. A major purpose was to get children to know and love their environment by observing their surroundings. The beautiful, the curious, and the unusual were often emphasized more than the understanding of scientific principles. Actual content included such aspects as field work, soils, aesthetics, farm and city locations and landscapes, building construction, economics, and politics. In addition, form, making and modeling, work with numbers, colors, drawings, and music were activity areas emphasized. There was emphasis on the out-of-doors, field trips, and plant and animal identification, measurement, comparisons, and representation of results. There was much concentration on aesthetic, emotional, and moral values.

Conservation education. The efforts and achievements of conservation education will not be detailed here, but mention of some major areas of attention seems appropriate. Content aspects have traditionally included soil, water, air, plant and animal identification, wildlife, and forestry. Other areas that have often been included are human resources, agriculture, rocks and minerals, space, energy, and basic ecology, including succession. Techniques of field-trip organization, sampling, collecting, and recording have commonly been taught.

Many organizations have been actively involved in conservation education over the years. State departments of natural resources, county soil and water conservation districts, and various park boards and commissions are often

Reprinted by permission from *The American Biology Teacher*, April 1971, pp. 220-225.
This paper was presented at the 1970 convention of NABT.

involved at the state and local levels. Other organizations are National Wildlife Federation, Nature Conservancy, National Aeronautics and Space Administration, National Audubon Society, National Park Service, Sierra Club, Soil Conservation Service, Tennessee Valley Authority, U.S. Atomic Energy Commission, U.S. Department of Agriculture, U.S. Forest Service, state departments of education, state game and wildlife commissions, state department s of conservation, and the Ozark Society. Often, private industries make free or inexpensive educational materials available, but the educator should be aware that these materials are likely to represent and promote the particular view of conservation that is suitable to the industry involved. The same can also be said, of course, about the various interest groups and governmental agencies listed above.

Outdoor laboratories and outdoor education. A clear-cut distinction cannot be made between current usage of the terms conservation education and outdoor education. It is possible, however, to suggest a distinction on the basis of overall goals. Conservation education has often focused extensively on the many content topics listed above, while outdoor education has been seen as education executed under the ideal conditions of the out-of-doors. Thus, the goal of outdoor education is to provide a learning climate (out-of-doors) which facilitates the achievement of various education objectives. Accordingly, the literature of outdoor education often deals with such aspects as management of an outdoor laboratory, programming, and the planning of grounds and facilities.

The content to be achieved may be similar to that described above for conservation education, but it often includes also objectives in the areas of language arts, industrial arts, music and art, social studies, mathematics, health, and physical education. Various individual programs also suggest affective (value, appreciations, etc.) and inquiry objectives in addition to the content areas already suggested.

Outdoor recreation. Camping, hiking, and Scouting are other outdoor educational endeavors often emphasized. Achievements include working together, preparation of temporary shelters, food preparation, helping one another, sharing and taking responsibility, and physical conditioning. Various other content and affective objectives may be incorporated as well.

Environmental education. Obviously, much of what is being attempted in environmental education is not new. At the same time, it is apparent that past efforts to generate favorable attitudes and behaviors toward the environment have not been particularly successful. Americans pollute and destroy their environment with little or no evidence of reluctance.

THE NEED FOR OBJECTIVES

The major objectives of nature study, conservation education, outdoor education, and outdoor recreation are not readily disputed. They continue to be

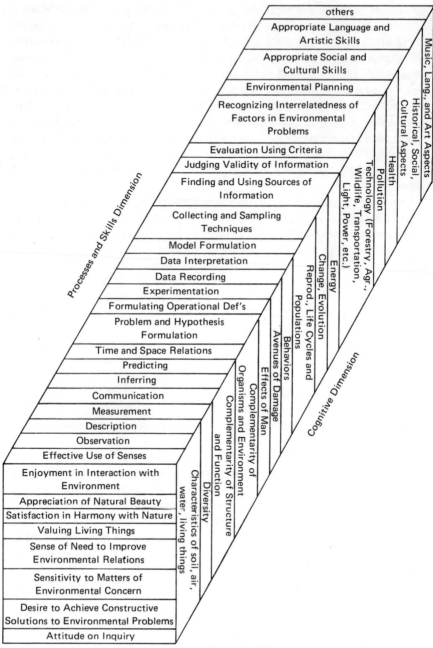

Figure 1. Grid suggesting some major areas of objectives in environmental education.

appropriate areas of concern. However, if environmental education is to become effective in changing behavior, objectives with behavioral foci will have to be developed. Curriculum development must then proceed in a manner compatible with these objectives, incorporating instructional strategies which develop behavioral changes. It appears, then, that environmental education must be an attempt to alter the behaviors of modern man by persuasion. There may be differences of opinion regarding the form this persuasion should take. Perhaps one individual will be persuaded on the basis of individual inquiry; perhaps another is persuaded on the basis of appreciations developed in contrasting environments. In any case, the individual is to be persuaded to behave in a manner less detrimental to, and more in harmony with, the environment than the past behaviors of modern man have been. We might expect these behaviors to be expressed in at least two forms: (i) behaviors implying concern about the effects of personal environmental destruction; and (ii) behaviors implying concern about the environmental destruction caused by others. Thus environmental education must be that which facilitates the achievement of such behaviors. As a science educator, I would say that such education should also be scientifically legitmate.

As those who have been involved in curriculum development can recognize, the specific behavioral objectives of environmental education will be very numerous. Behavior that is in harmony with the environment has many facets. Some of the areas of concern and behaviors are discussed in the next section.

AREA OF OBJECTIVES

In fig. 1 are shown some of the major areas of interest to the biology educator, in which behavioral objectives might be specified in environmental education. The activities and experiences of environmental education would constitute the volume of the grid and a given experience (visualized as being *within* the box) would normally have components in each of the three dimensions. In some cases, attitudes might be more heavily emphasized and in other cases one of the other dimensions might receive more attention. Such an encompassing view of objectives is appropriate if people learn individually and are persuaded individually through a variety of means.

A complete discussion of the grid is not possible here, but several features should be noted. Several of the unifying themes of BSCS (see E. Klinckman, ed., 1970: *Biology Teacher's Handbook,* 2nd ed., John Wiley & Sons, New York) appear to be particularly appropriate in environmental education and have been incorporated in the cognitive dimension. Second, various applications of our scientific knowledge must be incorporated if values concerning the environment are to be addressed, so technology is included in the cognitive dimension. Third, if we have the kind of faith in scientific inquiry that we usually claim to have, inquiry should be a major method used. Thus, various processes of science have been incorporated, including those of the process approach (see A. Livermore, 1964: "The process approach of the AAAS Commission on Science Education," *Journal of Research in Science Teaching* 11:271-282).

Certainly the grid of fig. 1 should not be seen as complete or final. The major emphasis here is on science, with various other curriculum areas only mentioned. As our understanding of environmental education develops, additions, deletions, or other modifications will be necessary. The point is that if the major behavioral outcomes described in the previous section are to be realized, decisions will need to be made regarding emphasis upon at least these three dimensions in the educational experience. Furthermore, activities considered should be analyzed to ascertain their strengths in these dimensions and to avoid a curriculum heavily imbalanced with respect to the dimensions.

Fig. 2 is an attempt to illustrate some of the major relationships of environmental education. At the center of the scheme are the individual and the environment, which interact as indicated. Associated with the individual are numerous areas of objectives within which behavioral examples can be specified. Also associated with the individual are the various types of activities in which he will be participating, thus gaining experience in the performance of the types of behaviors being specified. Associated with the environment are various areas of information with which the student will have experiences and in which cognitive behavioral objectives may be specified. Also associated with the environment are examples of educational techniques in terms of environmental setting. Specific behavioral objectives may also require behaviors integrating these two groups of objectives. The experiences themselves occur in an integrated manner.

ILLUSTRATIVE BEHAVIORAL OBJECTIVES

To illustrate, let us consider some specific examples.

1. For the primary grades, let us consider the following behavioral objective: "The child will respond enthusiastically and provide reasonable answers when asked what he enjoyed about the walk he and his classmates took through the woods."

2. For the intermediate grades, let us consider the following behavioral objective: "The child will spontaneously or voluntarily suggest the need to improve a situation, based upon his interpretation of data provided."

Behavioral objective #1 may deal with enjoyment in interaction with the environment, appreciation of natural beauty, or valuing living things (fig. 1). In any case, the affective dimension (attitudes) (#1) is represented. Though other concepts or knowledge might also be represented, the child will usually provide or imply characteristics of such features as soil, air, water, or living things, thus representing the cognitive dimension (knowledge, concepts). Typically, at least the processes of observation and description are represented in the achievement

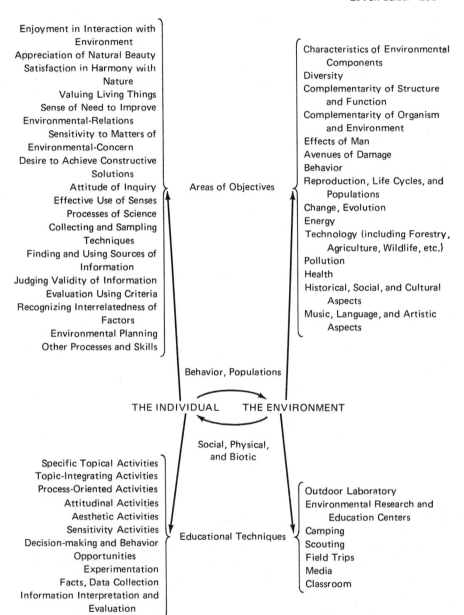

Figure 2. Preliminary scheme of major relationships involved in environmental education.

of this objective. To repeat for emphasis: the above does not suggest that all specific behavioral objectives will have equal components in all three dimensions of the grid (fig. 1); indeed, this would be unnecessarily difficult to accomplish. However, broad goals and specific objectives should be developed and implemented with an awareness and deliberate evaluative decision regarding all three dimensions in the curriculum.

The attitudes and processes described above are examples from the areas of objectives that describe the individual (fig. 2), and the information about the environment stated or implied by the individual partially describes the environment. (The behavior itself also partially describes the individual, of course, but the information conveyed pertains more directly to the environment than the individual in this case. The attitudes and processes conveyed, on the other hand, pertain more directly to the individual than the environment.) Quite likely the teacher would consider the activity to have an attitudinal, aesthetic, and sensitivity orientation, though it could be a combination of others as well. Facility-wise and environment-wise, it is a field trip, although it may also be taking place in an outdoor laboratory or other specifically designated facility.

It should be apparent in the example provided that there is an environmental influence upon the child through the social, physical, or biotic context that is provided. It is also clear that achievement of this specific objective is consistent with our overall goal of persuading the student to behave in a manner less detrimental to the environment, though the two are certainly not synonymous. This transfer of behaviors will continue to be difficult and much will continue to depend upon teacher strategies and behaviors. A bit more will be said about this later.

In the second behavioral objective provided above, the child provides evidence that he senses the need to improve environmental relations (fig. 1) and perhaps implies achievement of other areas of affective objectives. The knowledge or concepts reflected depend upon the nature of the data, of course, but population, pollution, effects of man, and "major applications" would all be fertile areas. Some of the processes likely involved would be inferring, predicting, problem-formulating, and, especially, interpretation of data. Attitudes, processes, and information can be related to the child and the environment (fig. 2) in much the same manner as in example #1. The activity would probably be topical and focus on information interpretation and evaluation (fig. 2). As described here, the activity could take place in the classroom.

ORGANIZATION OF CONTENT AND
LEARNING EXPERIENCES

A major goal of environmental education has been presented, and various subsumed areas of objectives within three dimensions have been suggested. The bases of these selections include such considerations as goals, student interest, and appropriateness, validity, and significance of content. Similarly, the organization of content and learning experiences must incorporate considerations such as child development, interest, logical structure of disciplines, the nature of learning, attitude development, facilities, social context, and teacher preparation. In actual curriculum development, such considerations are highly numerous and detailed. Furthermore, since curriculum development is a continuous process, content and organization will undergo more or less continuous change. Let us not be distracted here by the current hypothesis, however, that children should determine their own learning experiences. The potentiality for these experiences must still be provided at least in part through the curriculum; hence, a certain degree of structure and organization is needed for planning.

In the primary grades, considerations such as the following appear to be defensible:

Basic skills and processes of science (use of senses, measurement, etc.)
Characteristics of soil, air, water, organisms (observation, description)
Diversity (from obs., classif.)
Life Cycles (change, time relations)
Population (numbers, time)
Change (obs., inference, time relations)
Homes and habitats, needs
Gardening, foods
Weather, seasons
Behavior
Effects on man (obs., inf., likes, dislikes)
Avenues of damage (obs., inferences)
Pollution
Health
Enjoyment in interaction with environs
Valuing living things
Appreciation of natural beauty

Obviously, the above list is neither complete nor adequate. However, it should provide an overview of the kinds of areas in which specific behavioral objectives should be developed for the primary grades.

In the intermediate grades, the areas listed for the primary grades should be reinforced and deepened. Beyond these, the following areas of objectives should be emphasized:

Integrated processes of science (experimentation, model formulation, etc.)
Collecting and sampling techniques

Finding and using sources of information
Energy (light, heat, temperature, etc.)
Local changes, historical considerations
Complementarity of structure and function
Food webs (organism and environment)
Environmental factors and living things
Communities
Agriculture, food production, and simplicity
Forestry
Wildlife conservation
Satisfaction in harmony with nature
Attitude of inquiry
Sense of need to improve environmental relations

In the middle schools and junior high schools, many of the previously mentioned areas should again receive additional attention. The following additional areas or more specific examples within areas of objectives should be incorporated at the middle school level:

More complex instances using integrated processes of science
Greater independence in finding and using sources of information
Environmental changes, succession
Interaction
Ecosystems
Decision-making (local issues, committees, interest groups, etc.)
Health and medical considerations
Local cultural and social studies (special speakers, etc.)
Sensitivity to matters of environmental concern

In the high schools, much of the attention of environmental education must be given to experiences that will provide increased sophistication in the areas listed for the previous levels. In addition, considerable emphasis should be given to such areas as the following:

Evaluation using criteria
Judging validity of information
Recognizing interrelatedness of factors in environmental problems
Environmental planning
Desire to achieve constructive solutions to environmental problems

The areas of objectives as organized for the various school levels obviously should not be taken as mutually exclusive or strictly sequential. Evaluation as a skill will be taught before the high school, but it should be emphasized at the secondary level. Hence, the content of environmental education should not be seen as strictly sequenced, but an overall pattern does emerge. Needless to say, future experience may indicate a need for extensive modifications.

A few words should be said about the complexity and messy appearance of the environmental-education curriculum. First, we should attempt synthesis and simplifications of this proposal. Second, we should be prepared to accept that environmental-education-curriculum development that is specific enough to facilitate implementation may be highly complex. The problems of the environment and environmental education are highly complex and pervasive. This writer is impressed that the task before us in environmental education may well be the most important and the most difficult one we have ever faced.

COMMENTS CONCERNING IMPLEMENTATION

Environmental education should not be "tacked on" or added to the existing K-12 curriculum. My suggestions for environmental education in this paper are strongly science- (especially biology-) oriented, but simply increasing the science content is not the solution either. The entire curriculum must be infused by the activities that facilitate improving man's relation to the environment.

Irwin Slesnick, in a paper presented at the 1970 convention of NABT, illustrated a mechanism for accomplishing such infusion in the area of population education by bringing together various areas of the curriculum (such as art, social studies, health, science, etc.) on a grid. Space does not permit detailed treatment of this mechanism here, but this process must be carried out in environmental education. When the potential contributions of all these areas toward the ultimate behavioral goals of environmental education are worked out, we will be moving toward the total curriculum of environmental education in the K-12 span. In the process, we may even evolve some major themes around which our objectives can be more simply structured.